'People don't understand'
Children, young people and their families living with a hidden disability

Judith Cavet

SUPPORTED BY

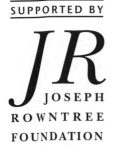

JR
JOSEPH
ROWNTREE
FOUNDATION

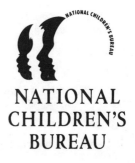

NATIONAL
CHILDREN'S
BUREAU

The National Children's Bureau (NCB) works to identify and promote the well-being and interests of all children and young people across every aspect of their lives.

It encourages professionals and policy makers to see the needs of the whole child and emphasises the importance of multidisciplinary, cross-agency partnerships. The NCB has adopted and works within the UN Convention on the Rights of the Child.

It collects and disseminates information about children and promotes good practice in children's services through research, policy and practice development, membership, publications, conferences, training and an extensive library and information service.

Several Councils and Fora are based at the NCB and contribute significantly to the breadth of its influence. It also works in partnership with Children in Scotland and Children in Wales and other voluntary organisations concerned for children and their families.

The **Joseph Rowntree Foundation** has supported this project as part of its programme of research and innovative development projects, which it hopes will be of value to policy makers and practitioners.

The views expressed in this book are those of the author and not necessarily those of the National Children's Bureau or the Joseph Rowntree Foundation.

ISBN 1 900990 24 5

Published by National Children's Bureau Enterprises Ltd, 8 Wakley Street, London EC1V 7QE

National Children's Bureau Enterprises Ltd is the trading company for the National Children's Bureau (Registered Charity number 258825).

Typeset by LaserScript Ltd, Mitcham, Surrey CR4 4NA

Printed and bound in the United Kingdom

Contents

Acknowledgements

This study was funded by the Joseph Rowntree Foundation. I would like to thank the staff of that organisation for their sustained support, interest and advice, especially Linda Ward and Claire Benjamin. I am very grateful to all members of the Advisory Group for the project who gave generously of their time and experience, including Patricia Sloper, Bryony Beresford, Priscilla Alderson, Leslie Prior, Edmund Kiely and Mary White. My thanks go also to Robinah Shah, whose involvement in the research broadened its perspective considerably.

In addition, Dot Lawton at the Social Policy Research Unit provided invaluable help in contacting families, while Wendy Sullivan and Jackie Clewlow at Staffordshire University made available unstinting clerical support. I am in the debt of all these people, and others who provided early and continuing support. Most importantly I wish to thank all those people who contributed information from a personal perspective, especially the families who participated in the research, speaking about a sensitive subject openly and eloquently.

Most of the families involved in this study were identified from the Family Fund Trust (then the Family Fund) database. The database holds details of families with one or more disabled children who have applied to it since 1973.

The Joseph Rowntree Foundation (which then administered the Family Fund on behalf of the Department of Health) provided access to the database, but the interpretations and views expressed in this report are those of the author and not necessarily those of the Foundation or of the Family Fund Trust, which is now an independent charity.

Summary

- This qualitative research with 35 families examines the social consequences of physically induced faecal incontinence for children and young people. Interviews were carried out with chief care-givers and their affected son or daughter. Their age range was eight to 22 years.
- The powerful social rules associated with this area of life meant that families faced public distaste, embarrassment, ridicule, general ignorance and very limited opportunities for discussion. The negative effect of this social climate was compounded by the invisibility of the condition and the pressures on all young people to conform to very narrow stereotypes of bodily perfection.
- Two children had achieved late continence. Nineteen used some special management procedure to manage their faecal incontinence. Parents and young people reported a boost in confidence when a satisfactory management technique was established. A clear and comprehensible strategy to achieve this end was needed. Families with the eldest sons and daughters were the worst served in this regard. Some were no longer in regular contact with a hospital and were unaware of recent developments.
- Parents wanted to provide their sons and daughters with opportunities equal to those available to other children and young people of the same age. This involved them in supplying extra support, both within the family home and outside it. Great discretion was needed on the part of all care-givers. Almost all families carefully limited the amount of information they gave out about the original impairment and its implications. Children and young people worked hard to conceal evidence of their incontinence. This resulted in significant emotional costs to the children and young people involved.

- Despite parents' love and concern for their children, there was evidence of severe friction in a minority of families as a result of the incontinence. The incidence of this and other secondary problems could have been reduced by improved service provision.
- Children were very largely educated in mainstream schools. However, gaining the provision of adequate social care to meet the needs of primary school children was often problematic. Individual support workers were highly valued by families, but as children grew older they wanted no arrangements which drew attention to their incontinence. Inquisitiveness and name-calling by other children was a very extensive problem, which could result in reluctance to attend school. Children required a sympathetic, supportive environment, with discreet staff and an anti-bullying ethos.
- Poverty was a factor in the life of many of the families participating in the study. The employment opportunities of the chief care-giver were constrained, and dealing with the incontinence resulted in significant costs. Delays in learning about relevant welfare benefits were frequently reported, as were inconsistencies in their allocation. A more proactive approach is needed as regards information about financial support.
- Further unmet information needs were reported. Families often lacked accurate information about the likely impact of their child's impairment. They needed to know the probable outcomes of surgery and whether alternative courses of action were possible, along with their advantages and disadvantages. Information was also sparse about how to carry out management techniques. As children grew older, questions arose about the implications of their condition for sexual activity and fertility. Overall, information which was honest, but positive in approach, was required in a variety of media and accessible language.
- National and regional children's hospitals played a key role in service provision, but local sources of professional support were very limited and require further development. In particular, general practitioners and health visitors need to be familiar with relevant information, and continence services have to be able to address the needs of incontinent school-age children and teenagers.

- The children and young people in the study were affected by a life-threatening condition and had experienced extensive physical and mental distress. The families' quality of life could have been improved markedly by a more coherent and relevant pattern of services provided to nationally consistent standards. Above all, a more accepting social climate would be beneficial. However, the children and young people interviewed were active members of society despite and because of the difficulties they had faced.

1. Introduction

Background

> Thence to my Barber Gervas's, who this day buries his child which he had lately; which it seems was born without a passage behind, so that it never voided anything in the week or fortnight that it hath been born. (Pepys, 25 July 1664, p 221)

This allusion in Pepys' diary refers to a child with a bowel impairment which affects about one child in every 5,000 born (Touloukian, 1969). As might be deduced from Pepys' diary entry, until very recent times most babies born with this condition were unlikely to survive. Nowadays, however, developments in modern medicine have improved survival rates very markedly, so that substantial numbers of affected children and young people live to adulthood. But, despite early surgical intervention, many of them are left with a significant degree of faecal incontinence as a result of their impairment. The condition which affected Barber Gervas's child is often known as 'imperforate anus'*. (For a brief description of this and other terms, see the Glossary at the end of the report. Terms which have been included are marked with an asterisk).

This study seeks to explore the experience of children and young people coping with faecal incontinence as the result of this physical impairment. It is also hoped that this research may raise issues which are relevant to young people coping with incontinence which is the result of other bowel conditions. Although rarely acknowledged, physical impairment of the bowel affects children and young people more commonly than is often supposed. It may be one aspect of complex syndromes like spina bifida*, or result from more specific and limited conditions, for example, Hirschsprung's Disease*.

Reasons for study

There has been relatively little research into this sensitive subject. My own interest in the impact of this and other types of bowel impairment began when one of my own children was affected, and I found very little information was available on the subject. It is already known that incontinence is a significant source of concern for young adults with spina bifida (Thomas, Bax and Smyth, 1989), but overall little work has been carried out which focuses specifically on this impairment. Reports of what work has been undertaken tend to have a medical emphasis. They are written for publication in specialist medical journals, and are therefore inaccessible to the lay person. Hence affected families, and those offering them formal and informal support, have few opportunities to find out how others have coped.

Information for a non-medical audience is required which addresses the broader impact of incontinence. This study therefore adopts what is often called a social model of disability (for further discussion, see Oliver, 1990), which distinguishes between the physical impairment which affects a person and any associated disability. The social model of disability proposes that it is social factors which determine the nature and extent of a person's disability. According to this view a disability is the disadvantage which results for a person with an impairment as a result of treatment by other members of society. This research seeks to explore the ways in which their environment affects children and young people with physically induced faecal incontinence.

There is evidence from those few studies which have been undertaken that faecal incontinence is very distressing to people affected by it. In the USA, Dittesheim and Templeton (1987) carried out a study which suggests that the quality of life in children over ten years of age is adversely affected if they are still soiling by that age. In this decade, three studies have been carried out, one in the USA (Ginn-Pease and others, 1991) and two in Europe (Diseth and others, 1994; Ludman, Spitz and Kiely, 1994), all of which indicate a tendency to emotional problems in children with congenital bowel impairment. These three studies used standardised scales to compare the behaviour of children with bowel impairment with that of non-disabled children.

Although these studies have the merit of drawing attention to the difficulties of children with faecal incontinence, there are some general problems with the methods used in this type of study. These have been noted by several authors and summarised by Eiser (1993). One drawback is that they fail to take into account the different circumstances which disabled children encounter. There is therefore need for a study which more fully takes into account the environment of affected children, young people and their families. This is because:

- Previous studies have tended to focus on the disabled individual and treat them and their families as though they are a problem, rather than concentrating on the social circumstances that influence their ways of coping and choices open to them.

- Even qualitative studies sometimes adopt an approach which inherently makes adverse comparisons between the behaviour of children with bowel impairment and non-disabled young people. For example, in the report of a recent qualitative study we read 'many of the boys and girls became overly dependent on their parents' (Ludman and Spitz, 1996, p 564). Thus value judgements are made without any discussion of deficits in availability of non-parental support.

- Little attention is paid to the pattern of service delivery, and the views of children and parents about what they want. One reason why this insight is necessary is so that formal and informal sources of support can be offered as effectively as possible, with the aim of avoiding the development of secondary problems and using scarce resources efficiently.

The research

Qualitative interviews were carried out with members of 35 families with affected sons or daughters aged from eight to 22 years. Most of the families were contacted with the help of the Family Fund Trust Database*. Children and chief care-givers were invited to give their views. Information about 14 girls and 21 boys is included in the study. Written consent was given by all children and young adults interviewed and by one of their parents. With the aim of including all constituent parts of the relevant population, families from all social classes and a variety of ethnic groups participated in the research. They lived in different areas of England and Wales, and had received treatment for their bowel impairment at about a dozen different hospitals. Half of the children and young people involved in the study were affected by an additional health condition. For more information about how the research was carried out and the people who contributed to it, see the Appendix.

With the aim of accurately reflecting the experience of the families participating in the study, this report contains many direct quotations, with an indication of the age of the relevant child or young person. The anonymity of participants has been protected by altering their names. The children and young people from families of Asian origin have retained names reflecting their cultural identity. The pseudonym of the son of the only family of African-Caribbean origin in the study is David. The reader can assume that the rest of the families were white. The ethnic and gender composition of the sample roughly reflects the ratio in which imperforate anus occurs in the population of the UK.

2. The social context: 'People don't understand' (*mother of Joel, 14 years*)

The characteristics and social status of the families contributing information for the research varied considerably. Some faced stress on account of lone parenthood, poverty or racism. Some were relatively privileged. Thus broader social issues compounded the disadvantage of some families and mitigated that faced by others. However, none of them were immune to the stigma attached to faecal incontinence.

Social pressures towards conformity to set standards of behaviour are particularly strong in regard to continence, especially faecal continence. Rules regarding continence vary across cultures, but all social groups expect control to be assumed quite early in childhood (Buchanan, 1992). Help with continence tends to be associated with infancy and perhaps extreme old age. While these social pressures have a generally functional aspect, they can produce a very negative impact on those who cannot conform to them. Thus an explicit consideration of public attitudes and people's reactions is a necessary starting point for a proper understanding of this condition.

Often these norms are so well learnt that they are taken for granted, and left unarticulated. However, they are key for affected children who are brought up in a world where incontinence provokes strong public reactions. This context has implications for their treatment by others and hence potentially for their own feelings of self-worth, as well as the pattern of service delivery.

Public distaste
'It's not very nice' (*Faith, 17 years*)

Public distaste for the mess and smells associated with faecal incontinence is deeply entrenched. Social pressures regarding cleanliness and odourlessness are probably stronger now than in the past, since modern technology and plumbing allows any manifestation to be rapidly obliterated, suppressed or disguised. Commercial interests employ advertising to high-light and reinforce the importance of personal hygiene for social acceptance. Non-adherence to accepted standards leads to feelings of severe discomfiture.

> 'She does worry about what people will think.' (*Mother of Faith, 17 years*)

> 'I feel it's dirty.' (*Farooq, 10 year old boy*)

> 'It's horrible. I wouldn't wish it on anyone.' (*Tracey, 16 years*)

Social rejection and ostracism can be one outcome of public distaste, and was a sanction experienced by some respondents and feared by others.

> 'I cannot take him to the mosque because of his condition. He can only say his prayers at home.' (*Father of Ahmed, 14 year old boy*)

> 'It was just like the stigma. Like "Smelly, I'm not sitting by him."' (*Mother of Colin, 8 years*)

Children too were well aware of the social effects of their impairment:

> 'Well, sometimes people just don't like me 'cos of me problem.' (*Patrick, 12 years*)

> 'People tease you and don't play with you because of this problem.' (*Nasreen, 10 year old girl*)

Awareness of public distaste for dealing with incontinence meant that parents, most often mothers, felt that they alone must carry out associated tasks until their child was sufficiently mature to take over responsibility for themselves. Few other people beyond partners and sometimes close kin could be expected to offer assistance.

> 'Not many'll volunteer. No one'll tackle it . . . no one wants to know.' (*Parent of Ian, 8 years*)

> 'I'm her mother; I've got to clean it up; it's me that's got to do it, the way I look at it.' (*Mother of Tracey, 16 years*)

This had implications for the independence of the affected children from their parents, and their ability to respond to opportunities to go on trips and holidays without parental support. One indication of mothers' awareness of general distaste was their particular gratitude to people who were prepared to accept and care for their child.

'They were smashing. They changed his nappy for him.' (*Mother of Stephen, 13 years, describing staff of his former nursery school*)

'He was really badly incontinent and it was all over the sheets and everywhere . . . He was covered in it. I mean, she weren't a bit, not a bit bothered! . . . I mean that's fantastic, isn't it?' (*Mother of Joshua, 11 years, discussing care given to her son by a family friend during an overnight stay*)

Lack of public discussion
'It's not the type of thing you broadcast' (*father of Jane, 14 years*)

Powerful social pressures exist which prevent the open discussion of faecal incontinence. The matter is not acknowledged in polite, adult society; and raising the subject is regarded as in very poor taste.

'You just do not talk about incontinence. You know, it doesn't come up over a glass of wine, does it?' (*Mother of Josephine, 12 years*)

'It's not a thing you go telling anybody.' (*Mother of Tracey, 16 years*)

This constraint on public discussion had implications for the ease with which families received and gave out information about their member's condition. It had an impact upon how open families could be.

'It's a difficult situation to tell people you're in.' (*Father of Jane, 14 years*)

'It's something people don't like to admit happens.' (*Mother of Karen, 12 years*)

This social rule which inhibits open discussion meant that even where parents wished to give out information about a child's impairment, they had to take care to do it 'delicately' (mother of Megan, 12 years), so as to avoid giving offence. Another result was 'a noticeable lack of people to talk to about it' (mother of Joel, 14 years). Full discussion was often limited to partners, and sometimes selected members of close kin. The need for trust and confidentiality was often highlighted as a prerequisite before any discussion could take place. The very private and personal nature of faecal incontinence was made explicit by some respondents.

'It's a private thing.' (*Mother of Colin, 8 years*)

Throughout the study, the need for privacy and sensitivity was emphasised. Children and young people often reiterated the need for discretion to be shown in the way any support is offered, since any public attention or discussion was unwanted. Pressures to conform to society's rules are so strong in this area that coming out against them is very difficult, and not an undertaking many young people in the study wanted to attempt.

Embarrassment
'People are embarrassed' (father of Phillip, 9 years)

Embarrassment was a reaction which was reported very extensively, both in other people and in respondents themselves. Young people and their parents put considerable effort and thought into ways of minimising the possibility of embarrassment. Fear of embarrassment could actually act to deter children from taking effective steps to manage the incontinence if the necessary action involved drawing attention to themselves.

Thus embarrassment operated very powerfully as far as young people were concerned. They also referred to stronger emotions like 'shame' and 'humiliation' when describing actual or potential incidents concerned with soiling.

'I don't think I'll forget that day as long as I live.' (*Simeon, 20 years, when describing an incident at his former junior school's sports day involving stained clothing and discovery by his peers*)

Ridicule
'They might have just made a mockery'
(Simeon, 20 years, explaining his need to keep his disability a secret from schoolfriends)

Humour tends to accompany any reference to faecal incontinence. Although joking about a subject has its positive aspects, it seems to be acceptable to poke fun at incontinence and its manifestations in a way which would not be considered appropriate as regards other conditions or disabilities. For example, a teeshirt exists printed with 'Colostomy's* not my bag'; and a fund-raising event for a national children's hospital included a joke about colostomy bags. Respondents drew attention to these tendencies, and viewed such humour as inappropriate.

'It's a nightmare, but to other people diarrhoea's funny.' (*Father of Phillip, 9 years*)

Children and young people feared being ridiculed by schoolmates, while parents too were mindful of this danger, citing it as one reason for limiting the amount of information they gave out.

'Otherwise they get the mickey taken out of them.' (*Father of Jane, 14 years*)

'My worst worry.' (*Thomas, 11 years, describing his fear of schoolmates' ridicule if they should discover his late gaining of continence and recent use of nappy liners*)

This concern was not without foundation. Many children had experienced ridicule and verbal abuse, as well as more gentle teasing. This is discussed in Chapters 4 and 6.

Invisible disability*
'He doesn't look like there's anything wrong with him' (*mother of Samuel, 13 years*)

People with faecal incontinence are not readily identifiable. There are no obvious, easily recognisable visual indications of their impairment.

'You wouldn't know there was anything wrong with him, unless you were told.' (*Mother of David, 16 years*)

'You wouldn't know, would you?' (*Teacher of Josephine, 12 years, on being reminded of her mother's earlier letter of information*)

The children and young people in the study were generally seen as non-disabled and often treated as such. While the invisibility of their disability was something which affected people and their families worked very hard to maintain, it did add an extra dimension of complexity to their interactions with others. One mother highlighted the situation with an anecdote about a cleaner's reaction to her taking her son into a lavatory for disabled people:

'And she looked at me and she looked at Stephen and she said "Do you know this is a disabled toilet?" I said "Do you know this is a disabled child?" And she looked at me, and I said "Well, I know he doesn't look disabled, but he is."' (*Mother of Stephen, 13 years*)

This lack of an easily recognisable disability had implications for the readiness with which access to formal and informal assistance was gained. While the effects of a child's condition were obvious to those living within the same household, members of the wider family might not be aware of difficulties faced, and therefore not offer support. Service providers who were assessing for eligibility for services were confronted with the same dilemma – they were faced with a child or young person who looked like others of the same age. Moreover, the extent and degree of any incapacity are not readily quantifiable. The following description of the reaction of a doctor who visited a family who had applied for Disability Living Allowance on the part of their son illustrates this point.

'The doctor said "Well so what? I used so many nappies for our little boy. What's the difference with yours?" And that's a local doctor who came, who's in the Health Centre now. He's still there, and he came and said "So what? We used so many nappies a day."' (*Mother of Colin, 8 years*)

The lack of an easy means of identification of a disability had consequences too for the way in which parents perceived their child's condition. They did not readily think of their child as a disabled person. This might delay an application for assistance.

'I didn't really think she would be eligible . . . You don't think of somebody with internal problems, like Faith's got.' (*Mother of Faith, 17 years, explaining a delay in application for Disability Living Allowance*)

More commonly, however, parents were simply not told about the availability of such benefits. This, too, was probably exacerbated by the lack of any visible indication of a physical impairment. (See Chapter 7 for a fuller discussion.)

Public ignorance
'They're just very unaware' (mother of Farooq, 10 years, of people generally)

Most people are ignorant about physical conditions which affect the lower digestive tract. Until their child's birth, most parents themselves had not heard of their son or daughter's impairment, and few had experience or knowledge of stoma* care. Lack of public knowledge and understanding meant families could not often expect an informed or receptive response from friends, bystanders or non-specialist service providers. This provided another disincentive to talking to people about their situation.

> 'I don't like telling anyone about myself because they don't understand.' (*Ahmed, 14 years*)

> 'People think you're lying, or you know . . . totally stupid!' (*Father of Phillip, 9 years*)

This lack of public awareness compounded the need for discretion if operating in a public or semi-public place. Privacy in changing even a baby or young child with a stoma is imperative if people are not to be shocked.

Many professionals too were lacking in knowledge and relevant experience. One professional response to this was to treat the child as something of a curiosity, thus discouraging parents from using local health facilities.

> 'They've never seen a baby with one, so he was constantly on show. Which is something else, I hated.' (*Mother of David, 16 years, describing reaction of staff at her local hospital to her baby son's colostomy*)

Some young people were very clear in their view that other people, including professionals, do not fully appreciate the impact of their impairment and its effects.

> 'People say that they understand and all these things, and they don't really, because they don't know what it's like.' (*Karen, 12 years*)

> 'You'd have to have the problem to fully know what it feels like.' (*Thomas, 11 years*)

Body image
'It stuck out on my stomach' (*Martin, 10 years, describing his colostomy and its acceptability*)

The prevalence and power of pressures to conform to certain valued body shapes is a well-recognised phenomenon in Western, industrialised society. Valued images are perhaps most narrow and stereotyped when applied to women and girls, but affect both sexes. Types of clothing worn can be seen as carrying connotations of maturity, desirability and conformity to group norms. For the children and young people in this study, considerations of body image enmeshed with concerns about their disability in two specific ways. Firstly they were concerned with the attractiveness of their bodies, and their acceptability to others, especially potential sexual partners. Secondly, they did not want their body shape to give out indications of their disability.

One illustration of these concerns arose in the children's references to the scars they had incurred as the result of often extensive abdominal surgery. Discussion of the impact of scarring from operations was partly about the extent to which it might be considered disfiguring. However, concerns were also about how to explain the origins and reasons for the scars which had commonly to be revealed in school changing rooms without giving out more information than was considered expedient.

Considerations of body shape and image were also relevant to the acceptability or otherwise of methods of physical management. Thus means of physical management were assessed for acceptability, partly as to whether they were considered unattractive, and partly as to whether they were discernible as an indication of incontinence. Colostomies were evaluated in this way, as were incontinence pads. Some children and young people found incontinence pads completely unacceptable. One concern was that their shape might show through trousers. Their connection with both babyhood and females meant that they were particularly objectionable to boys and young men, to whom the wearing of ordinary underwear was an important part of their image.

'Anything to wear underpants.' (*Mother of Stephen, 13 years, describing motivation for undertaking a further operation*)

Conclusion
'There's disabilities and disabilities' (*mother of Stephen, 13 years*)

The social climate associated with faecal incontinence involves public distaste, severely limited opportunities for discussion, embarrassment, ridicule, lack of recognition, ignorance and pressures to conform to very narrow standards of physical attractiveness. Parents frequently referred to this. Patrick's mother, for example, highlighted the negative impact of social attitudes:

> 'Colostomies and what, don't cause him a problem. The only thing that causes any problem is the outside world.' (*Mother of Patrick, 12 years*)

Some mothers noted that disabilities vary as regards their social acceptability, with faecal incontinence at the lower end of any hierarchy.

> 'There's disabilities and disabilities. This is a social problem.' (*Mother of Stephen, 13 years*)

> 'It's not like any other disability. It goes straight to the core of what the person is.' (*Mother of Joel, 14 years*)

This idea that being faecally incontinent is seen as a particularly negative attribute was supported by the fact that young people who were affected by other conditions were more likely to tell their friends about these than admit to incontinence.

Social factors explain why the children and young people in the study did not 'come out' about their bowel impairment and its implications. People very rarely admit to being faecally incontinent. Unlike most other disabilities, there are no public figures who are known to be affected by it. Families often put in a great deal of thought and effort to avoid the potential social consequences of faecal incontinence to their affected member. This is described in more detail in Chapter 4. A recognition of these social pressures is also important because it underlines the priority which needs to be given to achieving acceptable means of physical management. This is the subject of the next chapter.

3. Managing the physical effects: 'You find out as you go along, the best things to do' (*father of Phillip, 9 years*)

The children and young people whose families participated in this study underwent bowel surgery in infancy. Most had a colostomy in babyhood, which typically was reversed in an operation commonly known as a 'pull-through'* when the child was about one year of age. All of the children, whether or not their individual history fitted this general description, did not achieve faecal continence at the usual age. A key question facing maturing children and their families was how best to proceed in this situation. Specific advice was not usually available, and so trial and error might have to be adopted as the way forward.

Information and early management
'We just don't know. It's a matter of wait and see' (*mother of Joel, 14 years, describing doctors' advice regarding continence*)

Joel's mother described the circumstances after the reversal of her son's colostomy in the following way:

> 'They've got the back passage, but they can't make the muscle, can't make a sphincter* muscle, and obviously each case is different. They have to sort of play it by ear, the surgeon and the doctors. And they just say to you "Oh well, yes, he might become continent. We just don't know. It's a matter of wait and see." So you used to spend a hell of a lot of time with Joel in the toilet.' (*Mother of Joel, 14 years*)

Joel's mother proceeded with his surgeon's encouragement to put a lot of emphasis on toilet training, allied with dietary control and medication, in an unsuccessful attempt to help him achieve control. She went on:

> 'if they haven't got the equipment there, on the body, it's not going to work.' The result was 'Joel was always soiling.'

This sort of approach towards early management was typical of most of the children and young people in the study, in the sense that families were encouraged to pursue a prolonged period of toilet training which might need additional measures such as medication or dietary restrictions. These means had proved effective for one child in the study by the age of seven. Another child had become continent at ten, after further surgery. The rest of the young people in the study either coped with 'accidents' as a fairly frequent aspect of their lives, or had adopted a special means of continence management (outlined below).

Unlike Joel's mother, some families had been led to expect an eventual cure.

> 'I was under the illusion that eventually this problem would be sorted out.' (*Mother of Farooq, 10 year old boy*)

> '"I think you'll see a big change when he gets to seven." Then it got to be "Oh, you'll see major changes in him when he gets to ten years of age." So I don't know when the next step will be. I've not heard the next step yet!' (*Mother of Joshua, 11 years, describing information given by her son's hospital*)

Hence, families were often unclear about how much control would be achieved, and how soon. In the meantime, they found that both dietary management and medication could have their problems, as well as proving of limited effectiveness. In the case of medication, large amounts on a long-term basis might be needed to bring about any improvement. As children got older, further management measures were often introduced. Suppositories and enemas were commonly employed, and incontinence pads or sanitary towels replaced nappies as children matured. All of these means could be regarded as temporary palliatives until control was achieved, and were sometimes adopted with this assumption. Gradually, however, the need for more far-reaching measures became apparent. Bowel washouts* had been tried by a number of young people, and had been adopted as a daily routine by two teenage boys.

The mother of one of the young men said 'God, we couldn't live without it.' She went on to explain 'He's more in control now, whereas before he wasn't in control.' The adoption of an effective management technique resulted in changes in her son's behaviour:

'Since he's learned to do the washout, he's a totally different child. More outgoing, not so sort of withdrawn.' (*Mother of David, 16 years*)

Most of the other young people who tried this method of management had a less positive view, and ceased using the equipment or employed it only infrequently. This was sometimes because the method proved ineffective for them, and sometimes because they found it uncomfortable or inconvenient, or both. When the means outlined above proved unsatisfactory, some young people opted for further surgery in the search for effective management. One means of achieving this was to return to or retain a colostomy.

Long-term colostomies

Seven of the young people in the study had colostomies at the time of their interview. A couple of the younger girls had had colostomies since babyhood; one of their mothers remarked 'Well, as far as she knows, it's normal for her' (mother of Lucy, 8 years). Sometimes colostomies had been chosen as a method of management which was preferred to the incontinence which was the expected alternative. Occasionally the colostomy had been adopted because of medical complications. The children and young people with colostomies enjoyed active lifestyles and in their comments minimised the importance of their colostomy as a factor in their lives:

'It doesn't really matter.' (*Samuel, 13 years*)

'It doesn't mean much really.' (*Rebecca, 8 years*)

Some parents whose children had had long-term colostomies in the past also reported that these periods had been preferable to what had gone before:

'She was as happy as anything then.' (*Mother of Josephine, 12 years*)

This positive view was not shared by all those interviewed. For example, Susan (18 years) also described how she was 'over the moon' when she first had her colostomy carried out, since it meant the end of intrusive procedures carried out by others and resulted in more adequate management. However, she was hoping to move to a less obtrusive method, saying 'Some days I just wish I hadn't got it'. This was because of restrictions as regards clothing, outings, holidays and general independence from parents. A few other young people had declined the offer of a colostomy for similar reasons; they tended to believe they would lose opportunities they currently had – for example, to sunbathe on holiday or participate in contact sports.

The ACE* procedure
'The ACE procedure's really good news' (Josephine, 12 years)

Susan was in the course of treatment intended to allow her to use a relatively new management measure, called the ACE procedure. In this case, surgery is performed which allows washouts to be carried out via the abdominal wall. For Neville, the result of use of the ACE procedure was 'the first time he's ever been anywhere near clean for twenty-four hours' (mother of Neville, 12 years). Nine children and young people in the study were using this management technique regularly. Although it was not without its difficulties, views were very positive. It was seen by children and parents as offering greater freedom, security and independence.

'If I had the chance again, I'd take it.' (*Laura, 13 years, who also described the procedure as 'brilliant'*)

'It's changed his life. His life's pretty wonderful, compared to what it was before.' (*Mother of Stephen, 13 years, who had used a procedure similar to ACE for four years*)

One of the results of this improvement in management meant an increase in confidence for the children and young people involved. Both young people and their parents noted the change:

'She's more at ease with herself.' (*Mother of Laura, 13 years*)

'I'm more confident with other people . . . I'm more outgoing. I feel more confident with girls, as well.' (*Robert, 19 years*)

Intrusive procedures
'You get to a certain age and you're thinking "I don't want people doing this to me"' (Faith, 17 years)

The children and young people in the study had been subjected to a variety of intrusive procedures as a means of management, treatment or assessment. As they got older they often articulated their dislike of these procedures, for which their behaviour had indicated their distaste when they were younger.

In addition to the suppositories, enemas and bowel washouts already outlined, some children and young people, most frequently the girls, were distressed by internal examinations. Julie's mother (14 years) reported that from the age of about ten Julie would ask 'Do I have to? Do I have to?' about submitting to these on hospital visits. Jane (14 years) said of hospitals 'There's doctors poking you and I don't like it'.

A couple of parents had stopped doctors carrying out repeated internal examinations. Karen's mother was one of these and described her daughter's attitude as:

> 'No chance, you're not doing that to me when there's all them blokes standing round watching.' (*Mother of Karen, 12 year old girl*)

Boys were sometimes distressed in this way too. Phillip's father described hospital visits.

> 'I mean they're poking things up his bottom and all sorts . . . It's alright for them! . . . But you have to bring the child home . . . How do you explain to a two and a half, three year old kid that, what they're doing to him? . . . In the end, when we used to go to the _____, if the doctor went near him, he went off it. He knew! . . . he knew . . . In the end, I just said "I don't want you doing that".' (*Father of Phillip, 9 years*)

The most distressing procedure for many families was that of anal and vaginal dilatation*. The usual expectation regarding this technique was that parents would carry it out at home. Although some parents reported no problem in carrying it out, most found it very disturbing. Words like 'horrendous', 'traumatic' and 'abusive' were frequently used to describe it, and there was a good deal of evidence that children found it very painful.

> 'He used to beg and plead with me not to do it.' (*Mother of Patrick, 12 years, Merseyside, dilated until 10 years*)

> 'I just held the dilator in my hand, a metal bar about that long, and she, Sarah, just got up and ran for her life. Into her bedroom, shut, slammed the bedroom door shut and underneath the cot. And put a blanket over her head and wouldn't come out.' (*Mother*

of Sarah, 11 years, Midlands, describing dilation when aged about 3 years)

'My child cowered in a corner.' (*Mother of Reuben, 8 years, dilated when aged 3 years*)

Conclusion

Fourteen of the children and young people participating in the study had not gained continence, either naturally or with the aid of one of the measures described above. For some of them, this involved an element of choice. They might have decided that they did not want more operations, and that they preferred to use pads or deal with accidents. In the case of some of the children, especially the younger ones, families were still hoping that continence would eventually be achieved. It was by no means clear to them at what point these hopes should be dropped.

Some children and young people appeared to have slipped through the service system and to have few prospects of being offered a range of choices. There was evidence that the incontinence was a distressing aspect of their life and the importance of attaining an acceptable method of physical management should not be understated. For those still living with incontinence, their attitude was one of resignation, sometimes tinged with disappointment:

'You've just got to live with it, haven't you.' (*Mother of Joshua, 11 years*)

'I want to get rid of this problem. I won't, but I wish I could.' (*Tracey, 16 years*)

'We'll just plod on with what we've got. Because I don't feel she should be prodded about. I don't think she should be given promises that no one can keep.' (*Mother of Karen, 12 years*)

The general tenor of the interviews with the children and young people who had an effective management method was markedly more positive than for those without. Care-givers' interviews presented the same picture. The term 'colonic irrigation', with its positive connotations, was used with reference to bowel washouts and the ACE procedure, and parents of children using these techniques tended to feel their children were thriving. This sort of boost in morale has been noted with reference to other conditions, for example epilepsy and diabetes, when successful control has been achieved (Baldwin and Carlisle, 1994). This improvement in confidence highlights the need for a clear management strategy for all affected children and young people. Parents and children who had an acceptable method felt that a solution had been found and remembered the previous years as very difficult.

'It was a long nine years, a very long nine years.' (*Mother of Stephen, 13 years, looking back to the time before adequate management means was achieved*)

'Its rewarding end (that is, of a very difficult period) really is this big solution, this big miracle that has just made everything – it's so simple as well. The operation is so simple! And it is, it's so logical!' (*Robert, 19 years, regarding ACE procedure*)

4. Living with the emotional impact: 'They've got to live without it dominating' (*mother of Megan, 12 years*)

The challenge for children and parents was how to achieve the same sort of quality of life as the rest of the population while negotiating the possibility of the adverse public reactions outlined in Chapter 2 and managing the physical effects of the impairment in one of the ways described in Chapter 3. This chapter describes some of the stances families adopted and the means they employed to minimise the effects of the disability. The children wanted to be treated in the same way as other young people of the same age, and to 'live a normal life' (Laura, 13 year old girl, Merseyside). The overall aim of their families was to make available to their affected son or daughter as ordinary a life-style as possible, offering the same opportunities for fulfilment and enjoyment as were open to other young people of their culture and class.

Leading an active life-style
'You've got to live life to the fullest' (*mother of Joshua, 11 years*)

Children and young people participated in the great majority of everyday activities, including the usual leisure pastimes. The main area of significant restriction was in their freedom to stay away from home overnight independently of family support. However, this did not apply to all, and was most likely to affect younger children and those with a physical management procedure which demanded a disciplined routine. Overall families worked to reduce as far as possible the impact of the disability, so that children played sport and went swimming like their friends. Indeed, swimming seemed almost symbolic of this emphasis on activity, and the wish to lead the same sort of valued life-style as everyone else. Families frequently referred to it and the means by which it could be accomplished. Although it was the pastime where the child was most exposed to public scrutiny, children often wished to participate and were encouraged to do so by their parents, despite a certain tension being present.

> 'I remember the first time he went down to the pool, you know, and he'd be running out every three minutes . . . And, of course, he was running in to check. And he'd be out and he'd look up at me, 'cos I'd be sitting up, watching him, you know . . . And he'd say "It's alright!" (whispered). And he'd go back in and splash about for another three minutes! And he'd be running up to check (laughing), and he says "It's OK!" (whispered) and it was like a constant thing.' (*Mother of David, 16 years, recalling first attempts at swimming*)

Identification with non-disabled children
'He's always seen himself as normal' (*mother of Joel, 14 years*)

The children and young people did not think of themselves as disabled. Although they were dealing with the effects of their condition every day, some young people did not identify with notions of disability at all.

> 'Who's the disabled child? We haven't got a disabled child.' (*Mother of Karen, 12 years, describing her daughter's query regarding an application form for a disability benefit*)

Overall, most of the children and young people in the study lacked anyone with whom they could readily identify in an exact manner, because few had met anyone with the same condition as themselves, or been able to hear about their experiences.

Parents might tell their children they were 'special' or 'a bit different'; they might describe them as having health problems. Some children, especially those with some physical indication (for example, colostomy or ACE), recognised that they were different. However, the hidden nature of the children's disability meant many did not think of themselves as disabled. Where children and young people refused to admit their disability, parents were sometimes unsure quite what to make of their ways of coping.

> 'He knows there's something wrong, but he just refuses to accept that there's something wrong. So I don't know whether it's a good thing or a bad thing. So far it's been a good thing, 'cos it allows him to be very normal.' (*Mother of David, 16 years*)

'I think our Joshua tries to just, just push it under [the] carpet, as though it doesn't exist. But there again, why shouldn't he? He don't want to think about whether he's going to mess himself in the next five minutes, does he, or anything like that?' (*Mother of Joshua, 11 years*)

Information management
'Don't tell people unless it's appropriate' (*mother of Megan, 12 years*)

Given public reaction to faecal incontinence, children and parents had to decide how open to be about the subject and who should be informed. People who needed to know had to be informed in a way which minimised embarrassment to all parties. A key task was deciding who should be told. Teachers were informed, but children and young people frequently told none of their peers, or only one or two special, trusted friends.

'My two best friends know about my problem. All my teachers know, except for one. I don't tell my classmates because they would laugh. My best friend is very good. She understands and invites me to her birthday party. I won't tell anyone else because they will tell everyone and embarrass me and make me angry.' (*Nasreen, 10 years*)

Not all children could limit information circulating about them as effectively as this. Sometimes their condition became apparent, because of smell or other physical indicators. A few parents and teachers felt it was better to be open about the subject, and classmates were given a brief acknowledgement or explanation. The success of this strategy was very variable. Verbal abuse from junior school age children was a problem faced by many families, open or otherwise:

'They call me "beep pants" (I'm just cutting out the swearing). Is it all right if I go "beep"? . . . They always call me "shitty pants". They tell me to get lost.' (*Ian, 8 years*)

In these circumstances, the trustworthiness of confidantes was a matter which needed careful evaluation, especially given the volatile nature of children's friendships. Three girls had told one friend, from whom the information was dispersed throughout their class. The consequences for each were different. One who has an ACE found her classmates were interested and accepting, and she was in favour of their knowing because 'they can understand what you're going through' (Laura, 13 years). However, another girl who had no adequate management strategy found life impossible at school after disclosure and did not attend school for a long period. She remarked: 'Talk just gets everywhere' (Faith, 17 years).

Concealment
'What do you have to tell people for?' (Julie, 14 years, reported by her mother)

Because of the dangers of negative public reactions, children were sometimes keen that their parents strictly limit the circle to whom they gave information. Some disliked the idea that parents of their friends were aware of facts they might divulge to their son or daughter. Most of the children concealed evidence of the incontinence routinely and effectively. Continence pads, for example, were kept from the public gaze.

> 'Quick, put them in the car. They've got "Lady" on them.' (*Mother of Colin, 8 years, describing his behaviour when collecting pads*)

> 'He keeps his pads in his bedroom, but if his school friends are coming round I suddenly find them appearing in my bedroom.' (*Mother of Joel, 14 years*)

Children and young people covered any bodily signs of their condition so that they were not often discernible. Careful consideration was given to achieving an acceptable body image. Both boys and girls sometimes chose loose clothing to disguise pads, swollen abdomens or colostomy bags. Boys might wear baggy sweaters or football shirts. Girls had a wider range of options, although school uniform might require particular thought and adaptation. Adolescent girls and young women were under particular pressure to wear fashionable clothes which revealed, at least partially, parts of their body about which they felt insecure. The situation could become complex as several considerations affected the achievement of a satisfactory image.

> 'You know these little croppy tops they're into? She's sort of conscious of the clothes. Everything's geared round the top. It has to cover the scars. Pants have to be loose enough to cover the pad.' (*Mother of Karen, 12 years*)

Discretion also dictated that dark colours should be worn in case of accidents.

'She has to wear black a lot.' (*Mother of Sarah, 11 years*)

'Everything has to be dark . . . dark skirt, dark knickers, just in case.' (*Father of Jane, 14 years*)

'I used to love light coloured jeans . . . And I used to be gutted! I used to want these light coloured jeans and Mum said "No, you're best not having them".' (*Robert, 19 years*)

Some children very much feared discovery by their peer group, because of the sorts of reactions which might result. On occasions, especially in changing rooms and showers, some subterfuge was used to manage a difficult situation.

'I told them I had a kidney out.' (*Josephine, 12 years, explaining the scars to classmates*)

'I just say I've got a scar, so I can't go in the shower.' (*Samuel, 13 years, avoiding disclosing to schoolmates the fact that he has a colostomy*)

Not being able to be totally truthful placed children and young people in a difficult and stressful position. The dilemma that some faced was summarised by one boy:

'I was like, didn't want to tell them, but I didn't want to lie too much either.' (*Thomas, 11 years*)

Non-acknowledgement
'She just wants to pretend there's nothing the matter with her' (*mother of Sarah, 11 years*)

For some children, pretending their incontinence did not exist extended as far as their immediate family circle. Many of the children who had no clear physical indication of an impairment were reported by their parents to have a tendency to ignore and deny their incontinence at times, even within the family circle. This could happen in the face of clear indications to the contrary, usually in the form of smell. Parents sometimes referred to children 'blanking it out' or having a 'mental blockage'.

'He doesn't like it, and he won't admit that he's smelly, and he won't admit he's done owt in his underpants.' (*Father of Phillip, 9 years*)

Parents were at a loss to know how far the child really did not realise there was a problem, and how far they were refusing to acknowledge it. The same father said later:

'They do get lazy if you don't keep on at them about it – although partly he might not know he's doing it . . . know what I mean? And I'm not to say he's lying, when he says he doesn't know he's done it. How are we to know? . . . Unless you've gone through it?'

The idea that affected children had a tendency towards being 'lazy' was very frequently expressed by parents. This was as a result of children's reluctance to deal with the incontinence. This description applied to children without a clear management strategy and to some of those who had one, but disliked the self-discipline involved in carrying it out.

Conclusion
'It can be really emotionally trying' (Robert, 19 years)

The strategies developed by young people and their families were very much the logical outcome of the experience of social pressures relating to their bowel impairment. The way in which these influenced behaviour were also affected by the child's developing maturity. The child's understanding of their situation and condition was developing over time. One young man gave his view of the way in which a child's awareness and independence became established:

'From the age of zero to seven or eight . . . it doesn't really matter, 'cos you don't care anyway, 'cos you don't know what's going on . . . From age eight to thirteen is difficult . . . 'cos you know what's happening and you can't do a thing about it. From age thirteen to eighteen, you learn about it and you try to control it a bit more.' (Robert, 19 years)

Families put a great deal of effort into achieving as normal a life-style as possible for their affected young person. They were largely successful in accomplishing their aim. However, there was a cost to be paid if they were covering up an unpredictable pattern of incontinence for which no adequate management technique had been found.

'It does make you down sometimes. It can really upset you.' (Faith, 17 years)

'The saddest thing is being born . . . Why me?' (Ahmed, 14 years)

'I feel angry and sad and stuff.' (*Thomas, 11 years*)

For those children and young people who had satisfactory management techniques, their disability did not dominate their lives and their chief concerns were the same as their non-disabled peers. Others struggled to cover up their disability. Karen's behaviour summarises what could be involved:

'I mean I'll say to her "Karen, I think you need to go and change now". "I'm OK". And you can smell it! Or, if her friends come, she'll go upstairs and she might change the pad, but she won't get washed. Because she has to look like she's going the toilet, as a normal (and I mean inverted commas) "a normal child". So she has to, that's how it has to work. And it, it's – she sort of struggles. And she does struggle. Pretending that things are normal, she is normal, ordinary as well. She says "I'm just an ordinary girl".' (*Mother of Karen, 12 years*)

5. Family life:
'I want to give her all the opportunities in life'
(mother of Nasreen, 10 years)

Nasreen's mother's desire to maximise her daughter's life chances was common to all the parents interviewed. One challenge they faced was how to accomplish the practical tasks necessary, while minimising any negative impact on the family as a whole.

Mothers most frequently performed the physical acts of caring, cleaning and carrying out management procedures. However, several fathers also played an active role, either because they were single parents or at home as a result of unemployment. Fathers also carried out procedures their wives could not manage, or gave physical assistance where two people were required.

For some families, a female member of the extended family, usually a grandmother, provided an important physical and emotional resource, although not many were fortunate enough to have support like that described below.

'I think if Nanny hadn't taken it on board, I don't know how we'd have managed . . . Because they were brilliant, they did help us out an awful lot. Not only financially, in the early stages . . . 'Cos I mean with the colostomy and the nappies, we used to get so many spoiled clothes! And you could never get it out, could you! . . . So they helped out a lot with clothes, and they helped us out with nappies when we were buying them and Sandra would have nappies round at her house. If I called round I didn't have to remember to bring them and things like that. And then she would, you know, they've always taken them away and given them a lovely time.' (*Mother of Josephine, 12 years, of parents-in-law*)

Families' dual roles of caring for and protecting their child while preparing them for an adult, autonomous life-style are complicated when the child in question is disabled. The families participating in this study had to offer their child extra care and support, when necessary, while still encouraging moves towards independence. Some of the extra care took place within the home, including help with physical management, but additional parental support might also be needed outside the domestic environment if children were to participate in activities available to others. For example, where insufficient auxiliary support was available in a child's school parents might act as volunteers, or be available on an 'on call' basis. (This latter option seemed particularly necessary for children with colostomies, since extra exertion could lead to their bags becoming unstuck.) If school outings or swimming lessons posed a problem, some parents went along as a general helper so as to be able to offer discreet help, if necessary. This type of extra assistance was offered, while independence was also being fostered. Parents often signalled they were aware of the importance of self-reliance:

> 'I knew he couldn't make a meal ticket out of it.' (*Mother of Stephen, 13 years*)

Taking over responsibility
'Empty me bag out like a good lad' (*Ian, 8 years*)

One of the socialisation tasks undertaken by families is that of toilet training. Some of the families in the study faced a complex situation with reference to this role since it was not always clear what it was reasonable to expect of their child in this area. The task of training remained theirs, and yet they knew their son or daughter faced particular difficulties. However, the severity of these problems and how long they might endure had not been accurately specified to them. Faced with a lack of precise information, some parents took a gentle approach, while others were more forthright.

> 'We know it's accidents, so what about, as soon as you feel there's anything there, rush off and get changed. And we'll give you, you know, bags and things like that. You just get changed, because you don't want anybody else to know, do we? You know, it's our secret, isn't it?' (*Mother of Joshua, 11 years, preparing him for coping in secondary school*)

> 'They say "Will you get to the toilet, you stink!" . . . They'll tell him straight . . . And that's how I want it to be. In private – I do not say anything to him outside.' (*Father of Phillip, 9 years, describing older siblings' approach, endorsed by father*)

Those children who had adopted physical management techniques such as colostomies, ACE or bowel washouts, gradually acquired the skills and the confidence necessary for independence. Often the skills and knowledge preceded the confidence, so that children and young people might be reticent about taking over a procedure, even though they were very familiar with it.

> 'I think she could do it, but I don't think she wants to do it. Because I think that it's another stage in saying, you know, everything's not quite the norm.' (*Mother of Josephine, 12 years*)

Eventually, however, they assumed responsibility, although perhaps wanting the reassurance of knowing that their caregiver was within calling distance. Even when the skill was well learnt and always carried out independently of parents' support, young people often preferred the privacy of their own family setting for undertaking such procedures and had not reached the stage of carrying them out independently of family or special school support.

Family friction
'I've been really rough sometimes with her' (*mother of Tracey, 16 years*)

The anger and sadness reported by some children at the end of the previous chapter were also experienced by some of their parents, with obvious implications for their son or daughter. Issues of fault, blame and responsibility came up, especially as the child grew older and expectations changed. Parents were often at pains to emphasise to their child that their incontinence was not their fault:

> 'This isn't your fault, it's just one of those things that happens.' (*Mother of Colin, 8 years*)

However, some parents were not clear about what degree of control their son or daughter had, and how far they could be seen as to blame. They wanted their child to at least accept responsibility for keeping themselves and their environment in a socially acceptable state. Where children were coping by non-acknowledgement, this did not always happen. This led to expressions of anger and rejection by a few parents, all of whose children did not have an acceptable physical management technique available. Three families reported that they had been assigned social workers, following an episode of physical chastisement for incontinence.

Despite this parental anger, the children and young people in the study tended to take a positive view of their chief caregiver, describing them as the person who best understood their condition and the person who made them feel best about themselves. Parents were also the chief purveyors of information about their condition to the children, sometimes acting as interpreters of language and concepts which had been presented in too sophisticated a way for the children to understand.

Perhaps for these reasons, plus the fact that families, even with their shortcomings, provided a bulwark in a potentially hostile world, children and young people tended to feel it was good advice to avoid arguments with parents as far as possible. Parents were generally seen as allies whose support should be encouraged.

'I think really the only way you can stop yourself having arguments with your mum or your dad about it, is making sure you're doing something to help yourself . . . If you've had an accident, clean your underwear out straight away, then put it in the wash. Mm, because when I was a little bit younger, I made them mistakes, and that's what got my mum mad.' (*Faith, 17 years*)

Siblings
'I speak to Abdul when it hurts and I tell him not to tell anyone' (*Nasreen, 10 years*)

Parents sometimes worried that their other sons and daughters might have suffered as a result of their attention being directed towards their child with a bowel impairment. However, siblings were generally described by parents as helpful, caring and accepting of their brother's or sister's incontinence. Most of the young people who participated in the study were of the same opinion, although some felt that their siblings lacked real understanding of their situation. Brothers and sisters were supportive in a variety of ways. Some acted as confidantes, or offered emotional concern.

'They get all emotional like.' (*Mother of Laura, 13 years, describing Laura's sisters' attitude to her hospitalisations*)

Others helped with tasks associated with physical management, especially if parents were absent or needed assistance.
They also supported efforts at concealment, where this was
the way their sibling coped with their condition. They were
generally protective towards their sibling outside of the home,
providing physical or verbal defence.

> 'You've defended Neville, haven't you, sunshine, when people
> have said nasty things.' (*Mother of Neville, 12 years, addressing
> his twin brother*)

> 'He's very caring . . . They're just brothers. I mean he doesn't go
> round, twenty-four hours a day thinking of his problem. I mean
> he still fights him, and all that sort of thing. But he's very on the
> defensive. He's sort of – let's put it like this, he's sorted a couple of
> kids out once, that fought Stephen, kind of thing.' (*Mother of
> Stephen, 13 years, of older brother*)

However, younger siblings were less able to understand the
complexity of the situation fully. There was a danger that they
might be a potential source of disclosure or teasing, although
they were likely to risk parental admonishment in either
eventuality.

> 'He's got quite a big mouth so I wouldn't want to really explain
> things at the moment.' (*Faith, 17 years, describing 11 year old
> brother*)

> 'My sister used to be quite horrible, and used to call me "Holey".
> But I knew she was only little. She didn't mean it.' (*Josephine,
> 12 years*)

In general, however, the behaviour of siblings towards their
affected brother or sister was very much a reflection of the
family's methods of coping with the disability. Very young
siblings were uncritical and accepting, not having learnt
prevailing values. The unusual behaviour modelled in the
household might require some explanation and direction.

> 'Janet said "Why can't we wear them?" I said "You can't wear
> them, you're all right".' (*Mother of Julie, 14 years, discussing
> incontinence pads with younger daughter*)

> 'The baby's five and she's always seen Laura having enemas and
> stuff like that. But that's dead natural to the baby. She used to get
> the enemas and try and give her them! . . . When she was only
> little.' (*Mother of Laura, 13 years*)

Developing sexual relationships
'The right person'll understand' (*mother of Josephine, 12 years, reporting her daughter's view*)

The aspirations of the young people in the study as regards adulthood were the usual ones 'A job, a house, a girl' (Thomas, 11 years). Young people (and their parents) had often begun to consider and reflect on the implications of their bowel impairment for the development of sexual relationships. Sometimes they took a sanguine view, although it had yet to be put to the test:

> 'Because he's got so much about him as a person, that if they, if they fall in love with Joel then they'll just fall in love with the other bits.' (*Mother of Joel, 14 years*)

In so intimate an aspect of life, the means of physical management becomes an important factor of consideration. Joel, whose mother was quoted above, managed his incontinence by daily use of bowel washouts. An ACE is also unobtrusive visually:

> 'I'll just stick a plaster over it, you know. And the right person'll understand.' (*Josephine, 12 years, reported by mother*)

Some young people did feel inhibited to some degree by their incontinence. For example, a colostomy can pose problems as regards sexual exploration. One young person in the study who had a colostomy considered it an impediment to sexual activity, although it had improved her quality of life in other ways. This was one of the reasons she was undergoing treatment to replace the colostomy with an ACE.

> 'When it comes to the crunch, and she's gotta go with a lad – how she'll explain it to him, and what reaction she's going to get off other people . . . So I, that's, if the ACE works, it'll be like a dream come true. That's all I'm hoping for at the moment.' (*Father of Susan, 18 years*)

Four of the eldest young people in the study had experienced a relationship with a boyfriend or girlfriend which was sufficiently significant for them to entrust information about their condition to their partner. They only did this after much thought and reflection. In two cases only partial information was given. However, each had met with a sympathetic and understanding response. Although three of these relationships had subsequently broken down, this was for other reasons. The quality of the response to information about their condition remained important to the young person concerned.

'He just felt sorry for me. Just said "Come here love", and just give me a kiss' (*Tracey, 16 years*)

'I met her at fifteen. Mm, I actually slept with her at sixteen. And luckily the first time I ever slept with her, everything went absolutely perfect. Absolutely brilliant. And then, I told her. Because I knew that I were getting closer and closer to her. And that I'd have to tell her, 'cos if owt happened, I'd just die. I would not have known what to do or what to say. So I told her. And mm she understood everything. And everything carried on as healthy and normal as possible.' (*Robert, 19 years, who was keen to stress that he was lucky in this reaction. 'It could have gone totally the other way.'*)

Conclusion
'Don't molly coddle them, and try to make their life as normal as possible and let them do everything' (*mother of Reuben, 8 years, suggesting advice for parents with children with similar disability*)

Full social participation was the unanimous aspiration for the families providing information for the study. However, putting into operation the advice Reuben's mother expresses above was often very complex, time-consuming and stressful.

As families prepared their children for adult life, they faced many practical tasks and issues, and maturing young people tackled many hurdles. Responsibility for hygiene, washing and cleansing was gradually handed over to the young people, some of whom took it over with a degree of reluctance. Children acquired the skills necessary for physical management tasks, and gradually developed the self-discipline involved also. They sometimes grumbled a bit about the routine involved until they learnt and accepted its importance.

'He knows he cannot manage without it. I think once they realise that, then you're getting somewhere.' (*Mother of Stephen, 13 years*)

In addition to encouraging the developing autonomy of the young people in this and other intimate aspects of their lives, families routinely faced practical tasks which resulted in stress additional to that encountered by families of non-disabled children. Family holidays and trips still took place when sufficient funds were available. However, they required forward planning, attention to bathroom accommodation and the taking of copious supplies.

Families frequently overcame difficulties, but their workload was increased. For example, some families were living in overcrowded accommodation. Shared bedrooms and inadequate bathrooms were reported as exacerbating the difficulties of managing incontinence, and few families had received assistance in this area. The extent to which service provision acts to reduce stress to families with incontinent sons and daughters is examined in the following chapters.

6. School and work: 'The most difficult part of my life really was junior school and early secondary school' (*Robert, 19 years*)

Securing a supportive educational environment for an incontinent child or young person proved a complex task for many families. Although teaching staff were frequently sympathetic, important aspects of children's experience of school were not totally within their remit or control. Some of the issues which arose for families are described below, in the order in which they often occurred.

Gaining access to a suitable, acceptable school environment 'It was quite a battle and we were really worried' (*parents of Alex, now 12 years*)

As children reached school age, families faced two, often interrelated, hurdles when seeking to maximise their child's educational opportunities. First, they faced the question as to whether a school of their choice would accept their child. Second, there arose the question as to how the child's incontinence was to be managed in school and whether any assistance would be available.

All but two of the children and young people in the study could follow a standard curriculum delivered in the usual way. A few children did receive some extra academic input, but the general requirement of the young people in the study was a school environment which could accommodate their incontinence. The vast majority attended mainstream schools. Thirty children were pupils in mainstream schools throughout their time in education, two of these being in the private sector. Two teenage boys had spent their early years of education in special schools, before moving into mainstream. The three remaining young people were enrolled as pupils of special schools at the time they were interviewed, although one expected to move into mainstream in the near future. Two of these special school pupils had additional disabilities. The third young person disliked her special school and did not attend. With this one exception, families felt that the decision regarding the allocation of mainstream or special education had been made correctly.

The picture as regards availability of support for incontinent children entering school is very varied. The older teenagers and young adults in the study typically had started school without any assistance beyond that offered by their parents. They were generally expected to cope alone, although perhaps being allowed more leeway over being absent from the classroom. If there were major problems, a parent might be called in or the child would go home to wash and change.

Although the same measures were sometimes adopted with regards to the younger teenagers and the children in the study, this group were much more likely to receive, or to have received at some stage in their school career, physical assistance from someone employed to carry out this role. Table 6.1 demonstrates how the availability of assistance has improved. It seems reasonable to assume that these figures were influenced by the implementation of the 1981 Education Act. This law promoted the concept of integrated education, and improved the availability of resources to support disabled children in mainstream school.

Table 6.1: Pupils who were provided with assistance for incontinence during mainstream education

Age	Over 14 years	Under 14 years
Number with support	1	17
Number without support	9	5

Despite the predominance of mainstream education and the improvement in the availability of support for younger children, parents frequently reported a prolonged period of negotiation before a satisfactory outcome was achieved. Some felt they had to fight to gain access to mainstream education and adequate support.

A few families were fortunate, in that they found local schools which were able to provide a supportive environment to young, incontinent children within the resources they already had available.

'When I went to this school the head teacher was very good because her own daughter had problems with stunted growth. She said there was no problem: "Our five, six, seven, eight year olds still wet themselves and we clean them and they are normal children. This is a child who has got problems." She called her nursery teacher in who said there was no problem at all. We have never had a problem with the school; they are all very good.' (*Mother of Nasreen, now 10 years; this was the second school approached*)

Josephine's mother also tried more than one school before finding an environment she felt was suitable:

'So I shopped about, and we just got the littlest, little school on the estate. And they took her in nappies, and they were just brilliant. They really have been marvellous . . . They changed the nappies, emptied the bag, everything! You know, 'cos we went from nappies to a colostomy. They were brilliant . . . they used the poor old LSAs, you know. The learning support ladies, they – but they all made really good friends with her.' (*Mother of Josephine, now 12 years*)

Parents in both families quoted above were available to provide supplementary help on occasions. Nasreen's father was a school governor, and so could be available on school trips to help his daughter if necessary. Josephine's mother obtained a pager for the period when her daughter had a colostomy, so that she was always contactable in an emergency. However, both families were satisfied with the support available.

This was not the case for all families. Some children were accepted into mainstream school without the securing of resources to provide sufficient help or a situation which was viable in the longer term. Sometimes the demands such an arrangement placed on the chief care-giver, usually the mother, became unmanageable so that extra help had to be sought. This could prove a struggle.

'The fobbing off was unbelievable.' (*Mother of Stephen, 13 years, describing attempts to persuade the Local Education Authority to provide help in Stephen's school so that she could return to the job market, after her husband's death*)

'We had such a fight. It were unbelievable.' (*Mother of Joshua, 11 years, describing similar attempts necessitated by her own ill-health*)

Both Stephen and Joshua were eventually offered regular help on a peripatetic basis from a support worker based at a local special school. More formal arrangements were made for about 20 of the children who attended mainstream schools. These children had been issued with a Statement of Special Educational Need*, a procedure introduced by the 1981 Education Act. The result was the allocation of resources specifically for the child. Such a statement was sometimes the means of securing access to a local school with appropriate support. For some families, the multi-professional assessment process involved was unproblematic, although a last minute announcement of its outcome was not unusual. For others, they felt they were engaged in a fight. Jane's father described how he 'did battle with the local education authority and won', when the authority wanted to send his daughter to a school for children with severe learning disability. He gained support from Jane's consultant, plus legal advice, and eventually a statement was finally issued. Four year old Jane was able to attend the local school and receive auxiliary help.

> 'But, as I say, I was outnumbered fourteen to one. Nobody wanted her! Full stop. The headmistress at the local school didn't want her, the teachers didn't want her: but I did feel that there was a principle involved and that mentally she was a very alert, very normal child. And not to be disrespectful to other children, I don't see why a normal child should have gone into a school for children with special needs. Especially on a, on a mental basis then.' (*Father of Jane, now 14 years*)

Significance of help with incontinence
'At school I had to try and cope with meself, but sometimes it were – it were a bit hard to handle at times' (*Tracey, 16 years*)

Those children who were allocated a specific helper usually spoke of them with warmth and affection.

> 'She was a good friend. I still see her every now and again.' (*Thomas, 11 years, of ancillary helper in primary school*)

> 'She was nice. She was really kind.' (*Josephine, 12 years*)

Parents' experience was generally very similar:

> 'She were like another Grandma to him.' (*Mother of Joshua, 11 years*)

Only very occasionally were there problems, especially if the person appointed had difficulty in accepting incontinence.

'I don't think Mrs H would have held her hand without putting on surgical gloves.' (*Mother of Rebecca, 8 years*)

Rebecca's mother also indicated another aspect of the allocation of physical assistance to children in school. This was that she felt Rebecca was then labelled as 'one of Mrs H's children'.

If support were unavailable, then parents, usually mothers, had to be on call.

'I used to have to be at home for the phone call . . . I used to have to go up all the time . . . That's all that they did, just phone me all the time . . . And sometimes they didn't.' (*Mother of Susan, now 18 years, of primary school*)

Where teachers did not call in parents, but ignored the child's condition, the situation could be even more distressing for the child. Lucy's family were unusual, but not alone, in that they were without a telephone. If her colostomy needed attention she was sometimes sent home from school, or at other times left in school to 'wipe it off' (Lucy, 8 years). Her parents felt a leaking bag needed immediate attention, 'with the kids being so nasty, as well' (Lucy's mother).

The absence of physical assistance for incontinent children in primary school could prove very stressful to them. Tracey's experience (quoted in the heading to this section) echoes that of many of those without adequate support. Tracey's mother reported that she was called into school because:

'She were crying. She didn't want to do PE. She were really upset.'

David also had no help with the management of his condition in primary school. His mother explained that she had been very concerned about him coping with secondary school.

'Because he had such a terrible time in primary school, with the names, and my mother used to be going shopping, because the school was fairly local, and she'd be going past, and she'd see him standing in the corner of the playground on his own, and she'd end up in tears and everything, and we would end up in tears, and – it was tough, absolutely awful! Really, really bad for him. Terrible time. And then he started secondary school and it was the same thing.' (*Mother of David, 16 years*)

David's mother reported that the need to be available for him affected her employment prospects. The lack of ancillary support in school for primary age children had similar repercussions for other chief care-givers.

'I always had to be here. I couldn't go to work.' (*Mother of Laura, now 13 years, of time at primary school*)

'I were tied! You know, I was sending him to school, and I daren't go out, thinking if they ring me he's going to be at school, he's going to be messed up and I'm not there!' (*Mother of Martin, 10 years*)

Parents frequently needed to be available for swimming and school trips, unless ancillary help was available.

'Like they wouldn't even take her for days out, Chester Zoo and all that, when she was only little . . . 'Cos she was still in nappies. She was in nappies like, till she was seven . . . so they wouldn't take her nowhere. Wouldn't, wouldn't take the responsibility of changing nappies or, 'cos I used to have to go over in, at dinner time, and change her and that.' (*Mother of Laura, now 13 years, of primary school*)

Parents were often accepting of the fact that they needed to put in support. Phillip's father had given up work to care for his children after his wife left. He brought Phillip home for lunch each day to ensure he was clean. He said 'the school has been marvellous'. Phillip had no Statement of Special Educational Need; an auxiliary gave some help and called his father in, if necessary. Phillip reported he had been on school trips frequently:

'Sometimes for the whole day, sometimes just for two or three hours. My dad came with me. He used to come to the baths with the school, you know.' (*Phillip, 9 years*)

This type of unpaid help with faecal incontinence was rarely available from anyone, except close kin. These were usually parents, but otherwise siblings or grandmothers. Two middle class girls did each receive a limited amount of help from a volunteer, but this was very unusual. It is worth noting in this context that a Statement of Special Educational Need did not ensure that supplementary help from other sources would not be necessary. Some children were allocated half an hour or an hour of help per day. This could mean that they were left for long periods without assistance.

Dealing with curiosity and name-calling
'It were fair bad at junior school' (*Stephen, 13 years*)

The presence of support in school or the lack of it and resultant smell and other signals meant that classmates were likely to notice there was something different about the children in the study, although they were often not clear about the exact nature of the difference. One consequence of this was that children in junior school (and sometimes early secondary school) frequently reported being called abusive names, a phenomenon also referred to by their parents. This name-calling caused a great deal of distress, being described as 'vile' by one mother (of Sarah, 11 years).

> 'Sometimes boys can be very unkind; about five were horrible.' (*Rebecca, 8 years*)

> 'People keep, keep on making fun at me . . . say mm "wee bag" and stuff like that.' (*Lucy, 8 years*)

> 'It can really offend you. And it's not very nice at all, because you're thinking, "Well, I don't know that person, and they know such a . . . so much about me. And they're saying so nasty things." And it's just not very nice at all.' (*Faith, now 17 years, of name-calling during first year of secondary school*)

One element in explaining this behaviour was that the other children did not understand the situation.

> 'The other kids didn't really understand. I mean, sometimes now they say "You stink!" But it's only like not all the time, know what I mean?' (*Father of Phillip, 9 years*)

> 'People don't understand and, being so young, it's really hard to think of summat to say, and puts you on the spot and that. That was a very, very difficult time, junior school and lower secondary.' (*Robert, 19 years*)

The curiosity of other children could be difficult for young children to deal with. As Robert said, 'they were always noticing little things'. Some parents, children and teachers decided that the best approach to this situation was to explain matters.

> 'He had a bit of a stigma when people'd say, you know, like "He smells. Why does he smell?", or "You've pooed your pants" all the time. And then I just said that I think you should tell them. "Oh, I think you should tell them, that he is special and he shouldn't be laughed at. That's why Pat's there to, you know, is there to help." And they were great after that.' (*Mother of Colin, 8 years*)

Reuben's teacher also decided it would be better if some consequences of his disability were acknowledged to his classmates. She decided that they should be told soon after he started school, and persuaded his mother as to the wisdom of this.

> 'What I'll do is, I'll say, "Excuse me, this is Reuben, and Reuben wears nappies. Now you all know, you don't need to quiz about it, he wears nappies! So nobody's got to tell anybody anything, because they all know about it." And she did that, and there was never a problem.' (*Mother of Reuben, 8 years*)

However, Reuben's mother also reported elsewhere in the interview:

> 'They know Reuben is slightly different. They know he's got problems, because they know he's got his own room, and they know he's got somebody . . . So they do know something, but they don't really know what . . . And Reuben never really discusses it or talks about it. So, he gets a little bit of picking on and that, but I say, I just say, "Well, look, all kids get picked on about something".' (*Mother of Reuben, 8 years*)

Other families had also found that explaining the child's specific situation was only helpful so far. Stephen's mother, whose approach had been similar to that of Colin's mother, reported that the result was:

> 'They accepted him, but not always.' (*Mother of Stephen, now 13 years old, who elsewhere in the interview said of classmates 'They ridiculed him'*)

The mother of Neville explained his condition in detail to his classmates so that they were fully informed of his situation. This did not prevent name-calling:

> 'We tried to make sure that people understood why, but it didn't stop kids, did it, sunshine?' (*Mother of Neville, 12 years*)

New entrants to the class were one problem, but Neville's mother continued

> 'There's always going to be kids who, unfortunately, knowing other people's weaknesses will use them.'

Perhaps in recognition of this fact, most children and young people in the study did not follow the course of openness, but kept their condition a secret from most or all of their peers. Asked about how a school should treat a new pupil affected by incontinence, Ahmed replied:

'I don't think classmates should be told because they don't understand and for a new person coming to school they may feel very hurt inside.' (*Ahmed, 14 years*)

Growing up and moving on
'I aren't telling any of my mates at my new school now, 'cos – I just don't' (*Thomas, 11 years*)

The change to secondary school was a source of concern to families about to negotiate the move, being 'another hurdle to pass' (mother of Joshua, 11 years). It brought both positive and negative consequences. Secondary school offered more opportunities for anonymity and autonomy; on the other hand, the dissemination of relevant information to a large staff group could prove difficult.

'You can't explain to all, so many teachers.' (*Faith, 17 years*)

In some secondary schools this was overcome by issuing the young person with a card or letter which allowed them to leave the classroom immediately, without lengthy interrogation or explanations. Other measures which were utilised as a means of support included making available a special room (a facility also available in some primary schools) or arranging access to staff toilets. In some schools, a nurse was available who could offer support and take care of supplies of clothing and equipment. For a few pupils, a lockable cupboard had been made available. For the young people involved, the drawback to any of these measures was that they drew attention to their condition and caused questions from their classmates which they found embarrassing. Thus some of them might well not use facilities which had been installed or arranged for them. Pupils of secondary school were often very reluctant to use special toilets or visit a school nurse. Indeed, they might well find even the prospect of leaving the classroom with their schoolbag an embarrassing one.

'It's embarrassing taking your bag with you.' (*Megan, 12 years*)

'It would have been embarrassing to say "Wait a minute, let me get my bag and my pants and all this equipment".' (*Simeon, now 20 years, who did not carry supplies with him at school "Cos I didn't want anyone to see it or look in my bag or anything.'*)

For similar reasons, some children were unwilling to use incontinence pads.

'I'm not wearing them to school, the kids'll get even worse.' (*Sarah, 11 years, of incontinence pads*)

When asked what advice they would give to teachers about how to treat a child like them, the young people over-whelmingly indicated that they did not want any attention which would signal anything untoward to the other pupils. A general approach of not highlighting any differences was preferred. Asked how staff should treat a young person with faecal incontinence, a typical answer was:

'Well just that they're normal, like not to give them any special attention.' (*Josephine, 12 years*)

The young people felt that teachers should allow the children to leave the class whenever they wanted without comment. Secondary age pupils gave examples of behaviour in teachers which they disliked. Megan (12 years) who viewed some teachers as 'helpful, some unkind', found it unhelpful if the teacher said 'Oh, again' when asked for permission to go out of the room. A very common piece of specific advice to teachers about dealing with a child like themselves was:

'To let her go to the toilet when she wants to.' (*Tracey, 16 years*)

'You've got to give them total freedom in the bathroom, or showers, or whatever they need to do.' (*Robert, 19 years*)

Sometimes children looked back to their primary school-days and recalled examples of staff's behaviour they found difficult. The difficulty hinged on the fact that a teacher's behaviour drew attention to their difference.

'And he don't like anyone with a problem in his class. His class had to be spot on. Not, no one, nothing's wrong with anyone in that class. And, mm, he goes, just out of the blue, "Why d'you have to change in the toilets, Thomas?" And he damn well knew why. And I came out of school, and I cried my eyes out.' (*Thomas, 11 years*)

'I had this teacher who used to come into the classroom and say, "Karen, go to the toilet now", and all this, because she knew I had a problem . . . I felt upset, because it was supposed to be a secret and that's why she was my helper. Because it was just between her and me.' (*Karen, 12 years*)

Coping with a stressful environment
'And it gets you so upset you just don't want to go to school' (Faith, 17 years)

As well as managing their incontinence in the group setting of school and dealing with the curiosity and abuse of other children, children and young people were at an educational disadvantage throughout their school career because of missed schooling. This might be the frequent missing of small parts of the curriculum through having to go out of the classroom.

'He didn't want to miss out on what was going on in the lesson.' (*Mother of Patrick, 12 years, explaining reluctance to leave classroom and subsequent requests for teacher's attention*)

Or it might consist of breaks of several months for operations and other medical procedures.

'When I came back there I felt left out because like – I was away like for half the year . . . So I felt left out.' (*Samuel, 13 years, recalling effect of past hospitalisation*)

Some children were receiving extra help at school with academic work. Others were progressing extremely well, despite the stresses. However, for four children, the school environment became so stressful that they had ceased attending school for a lengthy period. Julie (14 years) who disliked her special school where she said she was bullied had not attended school for a year. Patrick (12 years) had missed a term's education by the time he was interviewed. Faith (17 years) and Martin (10 years) had also had lengthy periods of absence, but had returned to school after input from an Educational Welfare Officer. Martin's mother explained how the situation got unmanageable at his primary school. Although Martin was allowed to use the staff toilets to change, the clean clothing he had taken to school used to disappear by the time when he needed it. She would be called in repeatedly:

'And then it got really bad where the kids were really ridiculing him, and mm, they just had it in for our Martin at that school. He couldn't cope. He were near breakdown.'

She went on:

'Then it would get into little squabbles and fights. And there was only Martin getting chastised for it! . . . He was only defending himself.' (*Mother of Martin, 10 years*)

The situation improved for Martin after a new head was appointed in his school. For Faith, the switch to an all girls' school brought a much more congenial environment. There were indications that other children too sometimes preferred to withdraw from a stressful situation, either to a new school or temporarily to the safety of home, after an upsetting episode.

> 'He didn't actually go to school that much, 'cos it was easier to keep him off.' (*Mother of George, now 14 years, and a special school pupil, describing his period in the local primary school, to which 'I used to have to carry him to be honest.'*)

> 'Anyhow he was off school a week after that. He was so upset. He was really down, you know, over it.' (*Mother of Joshua, 11 years, reporting the aftermath of an incident of soiling when no auxiliary help was available due to sickness*)

Most of the pressures leading to this type of opting out were social ones imposed by other children. In Joshua's mother's words, 'He used to get a lot of grief from other children'. Affected children had developed a variety of strategies to deal with this, of which withdrawal was only one extreme example. Children reported employing firstly, bluff, plus ignoring taunts, secondly, attempting to distract attention in another direction, thirdly, appealing for help to a higher authority (usually teachers, but also parents, siblings or older pupils). They also used verbal retaliation, threats and finally, physical violence. (Only boys advocated or reported using this last measure.)

Some children and young people pointed to general factors in their environment which improved its supportiveness. These were additional to the use of specific resources, already discussed. They included the use of anti-bullying measures in some schools, resulting in an anti-bullying ethos which meant the children felt relatively safe. In addition, sometimes members of staff were particularly understanding or supportive, and this had a positive impact on the young people involved.

> 'But, mm, next year we're going to Belgium with school. And he said it'll be alright if I go . . . With me back and me belly.' (*Laura, 13 years, whose secondary school form teacher is encouraging her to go abroad on a school holiday*)

> 'He was real good, 'cos like no one can put up with me in a mood. But he did.' (*Thomas, 11 years, describing primary school teacher who tolerated him, difficult and depressed after traumatic surgery*)

Children did not want any special attention or favour from other pupils or staff:

'Just don't, don't be nasty, and don't be too nice. 'Cos it's not very nice when someone's so nice.' (*Thomas, 11 years*)

However, most of the small number of young people interviewed who had left school looked back over their school career and felt that a concerned and sensitive approach from staff had merit.

'Try and be as close to the student as you can. So he feels free to talk to you if he needs to, or tell you stuff.' (*Robert, 19 years*)

Adulthood and work
'And now I'm glad I've left school and got a job' (*Tracey, 16 years*)

Six young people in the study had left school. Four were in employment, one was about to go to university and one was undergoing a prolonged course of treatment.

The colleagues of the four young people in employment were unaware of their disability. The increased degree of autonomy which adult status offered and improvements in the young people's own ability to manage their condition meant that life at work was easier than it had been in the group settings of school.

Two of the young people had their own cars which also gave them more control over their environment than when they were dependent on public transport. Simeon (20 years) explained having a car 'is a massive help'. Previously, 'the trouble was worse, as I was walking to and from the station . . . and getting buses'.

Conclusion
'They've always been very, very good . . . They've never treated him as though he's any different' (*mother of Reuben, 8 years*)

Like Reuben's mother, children and parents overwhelmingly indicated they wanted equal treatment with other pupils by school staff. Nevertheless, for teachers to treat incontinent children as though they are not different from their non-disabled peers can be interpreted in two contradictory ways.

One view is that the child may be given the support needed for equal participation. Another interpretation is that it leads to the ignoring of a child's impairment and its implications. In Reuben's case, his school environment provided the appropriate help, facilities and privacy for him to participate in and enjoy the same activities as his classmates. However, for some other children, being treated in the same way as their peers meant being left to cope as best they could, largely dependent on their family's circumstances as to the availability of extra support, sometimes with distressing results. This was occasionally the result of parental preference. Two families did not want a Statement of Educational Need for their child. Parents were also aware that their child wanted no attention drawn to their disability.

> 'They treated him like I wanted him to be treated. They haven't made a fuss.' (*Mother of Joel, 14 years, who preferred this approach despite the fact that in earlier days 'he was always heavily soiled when he came in from school'*)

Staff attitudes were much more positive than those of pupils. Not all classmates were unkind, and some friends, especially close friends, were both accepting and supportive, but virtually every child in the study had experienced teasing and questioning which they found painful. Every child or young person interviewed wanted as little attention as possible drawn to their disability, and emphasised the need for discretion on the part of teachers. Yet to participate in school on equal terms, they required some sort of support, especially in their primary school years. Some children and their parents wanted more explanation to be given to classmates. Other young people wanted secrecy above all things. School staff have a delicate role to fulfil in this situation, and it is encouraging that 20 families took a positive or very positive view of the quality of staff support their son or daughter had received in school.

However, despite the goodwill demonstrated by many school staff, the availability of support within schools was patchy and appeared dependent on factors such as geography and extent of parental expectation and pressure. Assessments did not always appear to result in a just allocation of resources. An example comparing the circumstances of two eight year old girls living in different semi-rural areas highlights this point. Rebecca is academically able and has a colostomy; she is allocated one hour's help per day which is supplemented by her mother's availability on call, aided by a mobile telephone. Lucy is more disabled, having both a colostomy and a urostomy*. She is only allocated half an hour's help per day, and this is utilised to provide academic tuition. Both girls complained about their treatment by classmates. The support available to both Lucy and Rebecca was inadequate; in addition, its allocation was lacking in even-handedness and rationality. Quantitative research has already indicated significant geographical variability in resources available for supporting disabled children at school (Bibby and Lunt, 1996). The current study provides information about the hidden costs to children and their care-givers, both emotional and financial.

The locality in which families lived affected children's experience at school in an additional way. This related to how prevalent violence was within their school and neighbourhood, and the general level of fear of attack. This may have had a bearing on how open young people felt they could be about their disability, although it was verbal abuse which was the overwhelming problem.

There is a common theme which links the apparently disparate strategies children and care-givers adopted with regard to the school environment. This is a seeking for opportunities and respect, equal to those available to the rest of their age group. It may be that all pupils would benefit from being encouraged to consider more clearly their attitudes to disabled people, and to reflect upon the implications of acceptance of difference. These are important issues for inclusion in schools' curricula, especially perhaps in the light of the increasing numbers of disabled children being educated alongside their non-disabled peers.

7. Coping with the expense: 'Good God, how am I going to be able to afford this?' (*mother of Joshua, 11 years*)

It is well established that on average families of disabled children have lower incomes than families with non-disabled children (for example Bone and Meltzer, 1989). In preceding chapters of this report, there have been some clues as to why this tendency might affect families of children with a bowel impairment. These chiefly relate to constraints on the earning potential of the chief care-giver, especially when the child is young. Extra support from parents for incontinent children at home, in hospital, and sometimes at school, has an important impact on availability for paid employment. Because of the private and sensitive nature of the tasks associated with incontinence, delegation to non-family members is particularly problematic. Thus the employment prospects of care-givers may be adversely affected. Some informants indicated this in the previous chapter. In addition, in the longer term the earning potential of the young people themselves may also be adversely affected by the impact of missed schooling or the need for continuing medical treatment and further surgery.

This study was not designed to provide information about the income levels of the families involved. However, it did elicit a good deal of information about the poverty families were experiencing or had experienced in the past. Families without an adult wage earner were the worst affected. One example of former deprivation came from Tracey's mother, who described how she 'had it hard' when a young single parent, managing large amounts of soiled laundry without a washing machine:

> 'I needed a washer with a two year old, three year old when she had this "pull-through" done. So I mean I had to wash for five years, I were washing in the bath tub.' (*Mother of Tracey, now 16 years*)

For several families, bouts of unemployment of the chief wage earner made life difficult for a period:

'My husband wasn't working. He'd been made redundant. And we actually, we was, we were juggling between a pack of nappies and some meat for dinner, and things like this, you know.' (*Mother of Samuel, 13 years*)

There was also evidence of clear financial hardship affecting some families' present circumstances. Neither family quoted below had an income from an adult worker.

'When it comes to clothes and stuff, she can't buy them . . . You know, I mean, if, if she, the only time she ever buys clothes is if she buys catalogue stuff . . . And then, of course, it's paying for that.' (*Mother of Faith, 17 years*)

'They, mm, help us by putting so much in a fund every week, which means we have money for things like heating.' (*Mother of Neville, 12 years, speaking of extended family*)

Costs of incontinence
'Obviously they go through more pants, more sheets and blankets, and you know, the washing machine is constantly on' (*mother of Thomas, 11 years*)

The poverty which resulted for some families from their low income levels was exacerbated by the extra costs incurred by all families as a result of the incontinence. These costs arose for a variety of reasons. The amount of laundry resulting from incontinence was commented on frequently:

'I was washing, washing forever with her clothes, and sometimes I'd have to do them over again, 'cos as soon as I'd iron them, the smell used to hit me in the face when you're ironing.' (*Mother of Sarah, 11 years*)

'Bed sheets and his clothes and stuff have to be changed regularly, because no matter what, how you wash 'em that smell's still in 'em . . . You know what I mean? You can't get rid of it. Even when, like when you're ironing 'em, his clothes . . . Trousers and that, you can smell it on 'em . . . You can't get away from it . . . But you can't explain this.' (*Father of Phillip, 9 years*)

Moreover, soiled and stained clothing, bed linen and mattresses involved the need for frequent replacement.

'I've thrown away so many pairs of pants.' (*Mother of Joel, 14 years*)

'She's constantly in, in need, if you know what I mean . . . The clothes, underwear, bedding . . . It's money all the time.' (*Mother of Faith, 17 years*)

'You know, she's had that many beds, I've lost count.' (*Mother of Sarah, 11 years*)

Other significant costs which had to be met from families' incomes included travel (especially during periods of hospitalisation) and incontinence pads, when not supplied by the NHS. A major cost to some families of young children was the buying of disposable nappies for babies who constantly needed changing. In some areas a supply of free nappies is available for infants with bowel impairments, but most families had not qualified for a supply when their children's need was most acute.

'When he were born they told me it were best if Joshua wore disposable nappies. And I'm thinking: "Good God, how am I going to be able to afford this?" And this particular time me husband weren't working at all. I mean, obviously I weren't working and I'm thinking "How are I going to be able to afford this?" But me Aunty and me Uncle and me cousin, mm, they were absolutely fantastic. Bought every nappy I needed and everything like that.' (*Mother of Joshua, 11 years*)

'We just spent all our savings on nappies. Because this Health Authority here don't give you nappies till they're two and a half. So it was awful. 'Cos, like, I wasn't working and Mike was. And we just had to spend all our savings on nappies.' (*Mother of Colin, 8 years*)

'It was a lot of money out of what I was getting. But I couldn't, couldn't put in a claim for them, until he was four! . . . I mean that was scandalous . . . But there was nothing that could be done.' (*Father of Phillip, 9 years, discussing cost of disposable nappies*)

The strain of managing the additional costs of incontinence on a relatively low income was one which was indicated by care-givers frequently. Younger children tended to be shielded from the direct impact as far as possible. However Faith indicated how the financial pressures from incontinence affected her life.

'And it works out expensive in clothes. I mean I, I pay for my own clothes now. And I don't get paid very much because I'm still on the YTS . . . And I just can't afford it. I'm having to order clothes from catalogues and paying for it weekly . . . And underwear oh, and bedding! Well, my Mum pays for bedding, and she can't afford it. She's having to buy clothes and everything for my brother and sister . . . It's just really expensive! . . . And the hospital try and get you grants, but once you've spent it – it doesn't last long because you end up wrecking the things that you've spent that money on! And then you just need, you just need money all the time, constantly. Buying new underwear and bedding, clothes. Because sometimes . . . I have such bad accidents in the night I've stained my nightie, my bed, every-thing. I mean sometimes I need a new bed! Mattress! . . . So – it can get really bad sometimes, and you just don't know how to cope with it and I'm having to have baths all the time, and you know. I mean even that's wasting water, water bills and . . . Things like that. It's just money all the time . . . It's just a real pain.

And money to go places, because like if I walk somewhere or something, and I've had an accident I'm stuck . . . So – it's just a real pain, it really is. Sometimes I wonder how I cope myself. It's just, it just really is horrible.' (*Faith, 17 years*)

Gaining help with costs
'It's a bit of a lottery as to whether you find out about these things' (*father of Megan, 12 years*)

Given the extra costs of incontinence plus the negative effects of disability on family income levels, the availability of additional sources of finance is important to many families with an incontinent son or daughter. The families in the study had gradually discovered supplementary resources, although with varying degrees of ease and success.

Disability Living Allowance (DLA) is a non-means tested benefit which is available to disabled people. It is awarded to families of disabled children who need attention and/or supervision which is over and above that required by non-disabled children of the same age. Most of the children and young people in the study had been awarded DLA (or its predecessor, Attendance Allowance) for a period of time. In some cases the original application had been rejected, but the benefit was awarded after an appeal, which was accompanied by supporting evidence from professionals.

David's mother, who learnt about Attendance Allowance from another mother when her son was nine, described her experience:

'And when I did claim, they turned me down! They sent a doctor, to see me. The doctor came, he sat down. He asked David to go to the bathroom. He told David to get in the bath. David jumped in the bath, and he, er, says 'Can you come out?' And David put his hands on the side of the bath and jumped out, and he, he went away and said there was nothing wrong with this child.

And that got me really cross, and I appealed, and . . . you know, I said "Well I'm the one that lives with him. I'm the one that has to put up with all the, the mess and everything else, and you know, how dare you?" So we appealed, and the school were shocked. The, the, my GP. So I, I got the school, you know. The GP, and everybody else that we could to send in a letter, and the, the hospital as well, and that's when they decided "Yes", they would give us . . . the lower rate. And . . . they only could back date it for, I think it was eight months or a year they back dated it for, and for the rest of the time, we'd lost out!' (*Mother of David, 16 years*)

Those children and young people who were not in receipt of DLA were likely to be the older ones in the group and those without a specific management technique. Often those not in receipt of DLA fell into both groups. Faith, for example, now 17 years old, had never received the allowance, and a relatively recent application had been rejected, despite a very significant level of incontinence and resultant costs. Some of the young people had DLA withdrawn as they grew older.

'Because he turned round and said "Now she's old enough she can look after herself, you see. Wash herself down."' (*Mother of Tracey, now 16 years, concerning the doctor who examined her at 12 years*)

'They withdrew it because she was old enough to look after herself.' (*Mother of Julie, now 14 years old, whose benefit was withdrawn when she was 10 years, although she was considered in need of special schooling on account of her incontinence*)

Not all families accepted this withdrawal of DLA so phlegmatically, and some had challenged this type of decision successfully, with the supporting evidence from relevant professionals. The fact that some parents were less assertive than others about their child's entitlement to DLA was one factor in explaining why there appeared to be no clear relationship between receipt of DLA and the degree of incontinence families reported. Indeed, children and young people with techniques which had been introduced to them with the clear aim and effect of improving management were more likely to be in receipt of benefit than those without such a procedure. It may be that if a child had a colostomy or ACE then assessors felt reassured that a physical impairment did exist. On the other hand it seems ironic that the absence of helpful management procedures is not recognised as reinforcing the case for the allocation of the benefit.

The dissatisfaction which families most frequently reported about the DLA was the long delay which often had elapsed before they found out about it, and their eligibility for it, thus incurring very significant losses in entitlement. It was very common for families to conclude that they had lost several years' benefit. The general lack of information about entitlements was a major deficit in the pattern of services families experienced and is dealt with in more detail in the next section.

The contribution DLA could make to families was noted by some of the mothers whose children were in receipt of the benefit.

'For taxi fares, backwards and forwards and this, that and the other. And the extra bed linen, you know, just extras that I know, with having other children, I know how much he goes through clothes, compared to what they go through clothes.' (*Mother of Samuel, 13 years*)

'You can create diversions from the unpleasant bits. You can afford to take your children out for the day, which, if you didn't have that, you wouldn't be able to.' (*Mother of Joel, 14 years*)

Invalid Care Allowance (ICA) is a non-means tested benefit which can sometimes be claimed by a person of working age who is looking after someone in receipt of DLA. Only a small number of families reported that they were receiving ICA. Some did not qualify either because they were not in receipt of DLA, or only DLA paid at the lowest rate. In some cases the chief care-giver was earning more than the minimum sum allowed. More frequently, a parent was in receipt of a means tested benefit which they had been advised by staff at the Benefits Agency, or its forerunner the Department of Social Security, made a claim for ICA not worthwhile.

This rather glib advice may have been inaccurate as regards some of the families. The situation regarding the claiming of disability-related benefits is very complex, but only one family reported that they were receiving advice from a Welfare Rights Officer.

Information about financial and other entitlements
'Nobody's ever forthcoming . . . with anything' (*mother of Reuben, 8 years*)

No organisation was taking a proactive stance in informing these families of disabled children about the allowances available. This study indicates that families learnt about what might be available in a very haphazard way which they felt was disconcerting and highly unsatisfactory.

Karen's mother, who heard about DLA from a friend when her daughter was five, said:

'I think it's an awful lot for someone to tell you, just by chance.' (*Mother of Karen, now 12 years, who wondered what would have happened if she had been more secretive about her daughter's condition*)

Josephine's mother found out about entitlements when Josephine was referred to a London hospital for a second opinion when age 7 years:

'That was the first time we realised we didn't have to pay for nappies. Nobody had ever told us, or that there was disability allowance, or a carer's allowance for me, none of that. And that, that made me really angry. 'Cos we were only a young couple, and you know, we were really struggling for these nappies.' (*Mother of Josephine, now 12 years*)

These problems regarding the availability of timely, accurate and relevant information were compounded for the family for whom English was not their first language. Ahmed's family were assisted by a neighbour.

'He was an old man who knew my father. He told us we should get some money and he took us to the DSS. He was a saint. Without his help we would have had no money. Why don't people let us know that we can get help? I can't speak or write English very well and my wife is completely illiterate, so why do people ignore us?' (*Father of Ahmed, now 14 years*)

Hearing about DLA from an informal source in this way, usually a friend, neighbour or another parent, was the most common means by which families learnt about the benefit. Thirteen families discovered its existence like this, while seven were informed by social workers and three by health visitors (see Table 7.1).

Table 7.1:   Sources of information about Disability Living Allowance

Informal	Social Worker	Health Visitor	Nurse	Self-help Group	GP	DSS	Family Fund Trust
13	7	3	2	1	1	1	1

This delay in gaining information about DLA, plus the unsystematic means of relaying information about it, raises questions about whose role it is to disseminate news of benefits' existence and eligibility criteria. Although social workers were the professionals most likely to have broadcast this sort of information, families had contact with a social worker relatively rarely. The professionals who had routine contact at an earlier stage with all families were health visitors. Some families assumed that giving advice about entitlements should be part of a health visitor's role and saw any lack of information giving as a failure on their part:

'The health visitor never told me, you see.' (*Mother of Megan, now 12 years, explaining why her application for DLA was delayed until age 4 years*)

'She were lovely, don't get me wrong, but she never said a word!' (*Mother of Joshua, now 11 years*)

Occasionally a health visitor informed a family they were not eligible for DLA, and this resulted in lost benefit:

'It was only for the women at the hospital, you know, saying to me, "Go and claim it. You are entitled to it." 'Cos you think if your health visitor tells you something, they know best . . . Er, and I did. I got it, but I lost out on a few years because of them.' (*Mother of George, 14 years, who claimed when George was 8 years old*)

The other important source of financial help for the families in the study was the Family Fund Trust. The Family Fund Trust provides grants to families of severely disabled children on a means tested basis. The families in the study often volunteered information about the helpfulness and utility of this concrete form of assistance. Sometimes this threw light on the way financial help can reduce stress levels in families with a disabled child. For example, describing a caravan holiday paid for with Family Fund Trust support, one mother went on:

'And it does you a world of good just to have that break away, and come back again and you feel refreshed in everything. Because it does get a strain sometimes. I do get tired, you know . . . I mean it's no good saying I don't . . . I mean, I work twenty-six and a half hours in school, anyway . . . I do more than that anyway . . . You know, really, by the time I get home. I've got three other children, need just as much of my attention because I don't think they should miss out because of Samuel. So they're going to sports things, and doing this, that and the other. I'm running around with them, but I've still got to be there for Samuel in case he – even now. Even now he's older. I've got to be on call, in case he needs me . . . You know, 'cos I never know!' (*Mother of Samuel, 13 years*)

Information about the Family Fund Trust seemed rather less likely to have come to families through informal links, suggesting that the general public is less aware of its availability than DLA. However, it appeared to be allocated much more even-handedly than DLA, and parents were very positive about it.

Conclusion
'Nobody told me nothing' (*mother of Martin, 10 years*)

The delays and consequent losses incurred by many of these families before claiming assistance with the expenses associated with their child's incontinence were extensive. There may be several reasons for this. There were reservations about applying for help implied in some parents' statements. Nasreen's mother, for instance, was encouraged to apply for DLA by another mother who said:

'You're both working. You pay your taxes.' (*Mother of Nasreen, 10 years*)

Likewise, Stephen's mother spoke disapprovingly of some mothers' behaviour towards the disability benefits system, as she said they 'milked it'. She limited her applications, as did Phillip's father regarding the Family Fund Trust:

'But I never pestered 'em for clothes, or bedding and stuff like that.' (*Father of Phillip, 9 years*)

Another factor which may have been relevant to the delays was the invisibility of the disability, and the likelihood of its not being publicly acknowledged. In addition, in the early years there was often a lack of clarity about its permanence.

Nevertheless it would be difficult to disagree with Martin's mother's view.

> 'I think, if they knew it was going to be long term, I think they should sort of say, or somebody write to you for this, that: "You can get help here". But nothing! I've had to find everything off me own back.' (*Mother of Martin, 10 year old boy*)

The Benefits Agency does not take a proactive stance as regards informing families with a disabled child as to what is available. Local authorities rarely appeared to carry out this role effectively either, as far as the families in the study were concerned. Since the children in the study were affected by a congenital condition which manifested itself at birth, there seem few substantial reasons for such an unsystematic approach. As regards this particular condition, one outcome of the study is to be a leaflet for parents which will outline useful information, including possible sources of financial help, for dissemination by professionals and self-help groups.

The research evidence presented here is historical in that parents were describing experiences which happened some years ago, and it may be that the situation has improved. However, the indications are that a more proactive approach is needed on several fronts. Giving advice about welfare benefits is a complex undertaking and rules change frequently. Recourse to an expert may sometimes be necessary, but families first need to be alerted to their possible entitlement. The take-up rate by all families of disabled children could be improved by two measures:

- Local authorities are required to keep a register of disabled children (Children Act 1989). Supposing registers are compiled accurately and systematically, it would be possible to inform parents about sources of assistance at the time of registration.
- More training for health visitors about sources of financial assistance for families of disabled children and an emphasis on this approach as a preventive measure as regards stress, and potentially physical abuse.

8. Need for information: 'It's better knowing than like being kept in the dark' (*Thomas, 11 years*)

The previous chapter highlighted the importance to families of accessible information about sources of assistance with the costs resulting from incontinence. Financial support was only one area about which families needed to acquire knowledge. Families also needed to elicit and digest information directly concerning their child's impairment and ways of minimising its potentially negative impact. This was an ongoing process which developed in its focus and sophistication over time.

Most parents had to learn about the implications of their child's impairment very rapidly after its discovery, initially so that consent for surgery or other treatment could be secured. Mothers at this stage were still recovering from labour, and their affected child was frequently about to be transferred to a regional centre. It was perhaps for these reasons that information given by maternity hospitals tended to be broad-brush in approach, sometimes resting on a dubious assessment of the situation.

> 'They said to me "Oh, don't worry, 'cos normally it's just a matter of making an incision, and it'll be fine. You know, it's usually quite a simple operation."' (*Mother of David, now 16 years*)

> 'A lot of times it's just underneath, it's just a fine covering.' (*Mother of Stephen, 13 year old boy, describing what she was told initially about the extent of her son's impairment*)

Thus parents approached the regional centres to which their children were referred with a multiplicity of information needs, both immediate and longer term.

> 'I mean up to this point I didn't even know what the hell a colostomy was!' (*Mother of David, 16 years*)

> 'These things you don't really know about. And it's just absolutely devastating. I mean all these people are rushing in, saying "We've

got to do this, and we've got to do that, blah, blah, blah"... And the next thing you've got colostomy bags and dilating rods, and this and that, and you think "Good God!"' (*Mother of Reuben, 8 years*)

Role of Regional Centres as information givers
'They're good and that, don't get me wrong, but they don't tell you nothing' (*mother of George, 14 years*)

What knowledge and expertise there is about the management of physically induced faecal incontinence is largely to be found in the regional and national hospitals to which the children in this study were referred for their initial surgery. The key role of these centres in service provision is described and discussed further in the next chapter. From the point of view of the families' access to information about their child's condition, their personnel are major determinants of its accuracy, timeliness and accessibility.

Some families were very well served by consultants who communicated effectively with them.

> 'He was great ... He explains everything very clearly to you' (*Parents of Alex, 11 years*); and subsequently, 'I think he's really good, because he talks directly to Alex, more than he talks to us really.'

However, frustration was frequently expressed about the lack of accessible information concerning their child's condition, that is its cause, likely impact and means of management. Some parents felt that hospitals were unduly reticent about giving out relevant information. For example, despite finding the hospital 'quite helpful', Nasreen's mother felt the one drawback was that the consultant 'never gives the whole story at once'. Similarly, Laura's mother said of her daughter's consultant:

> 'He was a really nice man, but, he, every time you sort of asked him something, he just said "Oh, we'll just plod along with it ...". That was his only words: "We'll plod along, we'll just plod along". Never sort of, really goes, he never ever went into any detail.' (*Laura's mother, 13 years*)

There were several factors contributing to this common dissatisfaction. Children were under the overall charge of surgeons and this was the focus of activity and information-giving. Therefore surgery was often described to families in some detail, although not always in readily comprehensible terms. However, as the hurdle of initial surgery was passed and it became clear that the child's chances of survival were good, families' information needs became increasingly multi-faceted and forward looking.

Immediate information needs related to physical care; care-givers had to develop expertise in stoma care. Later, they were likely to need to acquire knowledge in other methods of physical management, for example, as regards dilatation, the ACE procedure or bowel washouts. Teaching of these techniques tended to be by demonstration only. Demonstrations were often brief, and there was frequently no supplementary information made available. This situation has improved recently with the introduction at several regional centres of specialist nurses who can offer ongoing advice and support. Up to this point, families were largely left to learn by trial and error, sometimes with negative consequences for the child in question.

> 'You don't know whether you doing the right thing.' (*Mother of Laura, 13 years*)

> 'Everything that we've sort of like done, we've found out when we've made a mistake . . . You know, it's just trial and error.' (*Mother of Colin, 8 years*)

As well as information about how best to provide for their child's immediate physical care, parents also needed other types of information. They were often unaware of the possibility of common complications occurring, until confronted by them after their child's discharge home. (The most frequently reported scenario related to prolapsing of stomas, which could be alarming for parents who had not been forewarned.) Other information, pertaining to medical or nursing procedures and not routinely given, related to how successful the pull-through operation was likely to be in terms of achievement of continence. Parents did not always know the right questions to ask in order to elicit significant information, and doctors seemed unlikely to volunteer it. With hindsight, some parents regretted having the pull-through operation carried out because of ensuing physical and psychological distress for their child. However, not attempting the 'pull-through' had not usually been acknowledged as a course which might be chosen, rather than imposed by additional medical considerations.

Thus families needed information which made clear the likely impact of surgical interventions. Minimising the probable effects of the impairment was unhelpful as it misled families about what it was reasonable to expect of their child in terms of continence. This lack of clarity could lead to the anger noted in Chapter 4. Frustration and occasional violence might have been avoided if more accurate information was made available. The quotation below makes these links and demonstrates how punitive or rejecting attitudes could develop.

Tracey's mother described how she had lost her temper with her daughter after a particularly messy bout of incontinence and smacked her so hard that 'I'd left handprints on her bum'. Subsequently:

> 'I went to hospital and I saw a doctor there and I says "All I want is a simple answer. Can she help it, or can't she help it? 'Cos the answer I keep getting is 'Yes she can'. 'No, she can't'!" So I said "I want a simple answer". And I got the same answer when I went, so it were a waste of time.' (*Mother of Tracey, now 16 years, of an incident which took place at age 8 or 9 years*)

In these circumstances it is difficult to disagree with Haroon's mother:

> 'I think the doctors should be more honest about the future. We were led to believe that after the pull-through he would be perfectly "normal".' (*Mother of Haroon, now 22 years*)

Another area where it would be valuable for families to have an acknowledgement of, perhaps unpalatable, facts relates to the invasive procedures parents are expected to carry out and children accept. A recognition of the disturbing and distressing nature of procedures like anal dilatation would be useful for families. It is also important to note that children and young people were regularly being subjected to invasive procedures which in other circumstances would be illegal. Those responsible for initiating such procedures need to be very clear that any potential gain warrants the damaging consequences for the children involved.

Information needs altered as children developed and matured, and as knowledge and techniques changed. Moreover, parents of older children and sometimes the young people themselves had queries about fertility and sexual activity which were relevant to teenagers and which were unlikely to have been approached earlier. Few consultants had dealt with this question as explicitly as Josephine's:

'When you're ready to have sex, you give me a ring and we'll sort it out.' (*Reported by mother of Josephine, 12 years*)

More information is needed for parents
'Better educated parents to educate the kids' (*father of Phillip, 9 years*)

Parents required full information in order to provide good quality physical care for their child and in order to make informed decisions about further surgery and other treatments. They also needed to be as informed as possible about the likely impact on their child's future development in order to provide an appropriate environment. Part of their role was as providers of information about their child's condition to people who needed this knowledge. Foremost among those needing to know were the children themselves. Parents were the chief source of information for their children as regards the nature of their condition, its likely impact and most suitable means of managing it. This reinforces the need for parents to have access to adequate information.

'The only information has come from me . . . and I only know the basics of it.' (*Father of Jane, 14 years*)

'Well, my mum tells me everything and the doctors don't say anything to me!' (*Lucy, 8 years*)

While some doctors did communicate directly with their patients, even in these families parents were important sources of information for children so that the resources spent in enhancing parental understanding were worthwhile.

Understanding the causes
'I want to know what causes it me' (*Tracey, 16 years*)

One major frustration for families was that very little information is available about causation, probably a result of research interest (and funding) reflecting the public distaste. Some parents were given simplistic explanations.

'All we were told was "It's just one of them things" . . . which is not good enough.' (*Parents of Lucy, 8 years*)

'It was a bad egg.' (*Mother of Karen, 12 years, repeating the explanation she was offered*)

'"Oh, it's just one of those things. It's unfortunate that it's happened to you twice". And I thought, you know, (small laugh), you know, this is a bit – offish, like, you know.' (*Mother of Thomas, 11 years, describing information proffered after the birth of her second affected child*)

This lack of an adequate explanation meant that the children's frequent question 'Why me?' was very difficult to answer, even at the level of straight information.

'It is difficult, and the age he's at he doesn't understand much of what I'm trying to say to him, he just wants a straight answer "why" and there is no real reason.' (*Mother of Farooq, 10 years*)

'She needs to be told a bit more like, for her to understand why, you know, she's had to have a colostomy.' (*Parents of Lucy, 8 years*)

Information for children
'It was me who was having the operation, not my Dad' (*Thomas, 11 years*)

As regards availability of information for children and young people, there were broadly three overlapping groups of children spread along a continuum of knowledgeability. Firstly there were those children who were provided with information by one or both parents, plus their consultant. Where consultants were skilled at communicating directly with children, of different ages and levels of maturity, children had a clear grasp of the cause of their disability, and the course of medical input. Angela (8 years) who said that 'Mummy and Mr G' explained her disability to her could report pithily 'I was born without a bumhole'. Asked about her condition, Josephine (12 years) described her medical history:

'I had my kidney out when I was little, and then I had to keep going back, 'cos I had a colostomy and then I had the ACE procedure, and yeah, I've had that about two years, I think.'

Asked about where her information came from she reported input from her mother and her consultant:

'He tried to explain and he drew pictures, but it was quite hard. But my mum was a nurse before, so she understood it better.' (*Josephine, 12 years*)

Secondly, there were children and young people whose parents were their only direct source of information. In this case, doctors spoke only to the parents who acted as interpreters and communicators. Parents and children were often somewhat less satisfied with this system because of the child's exclusion from an exchange in which they were the key person. The system also worked badly if parents did not themselves understand a situation or treatment rationale, or if they were not available to support their child because of other caring commitments.

> 'He's sat there with me but it's like through me. "Does he go to the toilet, does he do this, does he do that?" And when they get to nine and ten, they can answer theirself, easy . . . I mean he could up from five . . . 'Cos there's no flies on that kid!' (*Father of Phillip, 9 years*)

> 'He's sitting there and they talk about him as though he's not there. Mm, and while they're talking about him, we're saying "Do you know that, George?" You know, we try and include him into it . . . 'cos we're talking about George, we go, we look at George and we're both talking to George and the specialist together. But they don't. They only ever talk to us.' (*Mother of George, 14 years*)

George may have been particularly badly served by the medical profession as regards communication for a number of related reasons which to some degree affected adversely the interactions of other children and young people with their doctors. One important barrier was social class. George perceived his doctors as 'dead posh', and described in his interview how he sought to avoid contact with them if he was alone. There were some indications that he and his family found discussions with his consultant potentially intimidating. George's educational level and attendance at a special school may have reinforced lack of ease on both sides of the communication. A few parents noted the discomfort of their children in discussions with consultants. This was partly perhaps due to factors already noted, compounded by embarrassment or the wish to avoid any overt recognition of the incontinence.

Despite this possible discomfiture, most children and young people wanted information aimed at them directly. Samuel explained:

> 'Mum usually tells me, like, you know, when I'm going in . . . Doctor tells her and Mum tells me. So what's going to happen and all that. He doesn't tell you (i.e. me).' (*Samuel, 13 years*)

Although Samuel was kept well informed by his mother, he stated subsequently he wanted his doctors to tell him 'exactly what's going to happen' on his admissions to hospital.

On those infrequent but unavoidable occasions where parents could not provide a liaison between doctors and children, hospital admissions could prove very distressing if doctors did not explain the rationale for a treatment regime. Thomas was very dissatisfied with communication about an operation carried out when he was ten. He had no idea of why the operation was performed.

> 'They could explain what they were going to do, to me, not my Dad. I mean, it was me who was having the operation, not my Dad.' (*Thomas, 11 years*)

He wanted information about the rationale for surgery and for any drugs administered. He also wanted accurate information about the amount of pain to expect. He said strongly 'They just told me a pack of lies'. An example of this being 'Oh, this won't hurt'.

Faith, too, had no idea of the reason for one lengthy hospital admission, in this case to 'a very strict ward':

> 'I mean they never did anything special to me . . . I was just in there for three months for no reason'; and later, 'I don't know why they did it, I really don't.' (*Faith, now 17 years, of hospital stay when aged 11*)

Despite these deficits in their knowledge, both Thomas and Faith did know the physical origins of their disability. However, some young people displayed a lack of familiarity which was disconcerting given their relative maturity. This third group were the worst served as regards information and their knowledge base was very limited. This group of young people was no longer receiving regular medical input.

> 'All I've been told is that I've got a problem with my bowel and I can't hold things in. That's all I've been told. Haven't been told why, or what caused it, or anything like that.' (*Karen, 12 years*)

> 'All me Mum said: like, I've got a hole in my heart and everything and that, and I'd got no back passage, and that were it. That's all she's ever said to me.' (*Tracey, 16 years*)

> 'My operation was at the back. Why have I got stitches at the front? I don't understand that part.' (*Jane, 14 years*)

Learning from others in the same position
'I used to think there was no one who had the same problem as me' (Karen, 12 years)

Several parents and children reported that they had been under the impression for a lengthy period that they were the only families affected by their condition. The most common way that they were disabused of this idea was by meetings in the regional hospitals. Such encounters were usually informal and by chance, but the source of much useful information and support. In addition, staff at a couple of regional hospitals had organised parties for affected children, and in this case both parents and children could meet others in a similar position. These opportunities were valued:

> 'We don't really talk about the operation, we just enjoy ourselves while we're there, but it's quite – it's really fun.' (*Josephine, 12 years*)

A small number of young people had been introduced to a child or teenager with relevant experience in order to learn their views about an unfamiliar management technique they were considering adopting. Their parents too sometimes met to exchange information. These opportunities were organised by hospital staff and perceived as useful. All those young people who had met a person with a similar condition were positive about the experience. Several, though not all, of secondary school age children who had not done so, also felt there were likely to be potential benefits. In general, all these types of contact helped to reduce isolation and there was scope for further development. Susan and her parents would have liked to discuss stoma care with someone of a similar age who lived in their locality:

> 'You think you're the only one. You don't realise there is quite a few other people.' (*Mother of Susan, 18 years*)

Nationally-based self-help groups* did not play a major role as regards information provision for the families participating in the study. Only a small number of families were aware of the existence of such groups. Even fewer had contacted a self-help group, although those who had had discovered useful information about the wider pattern of service provision.

Paucity of written information
'I got nothing. Zero. Absolutely zero' (mother of Reuben, 8 years)

The discussion of information availability has concentrated so far on oral information only. This is because so little written information is available to the interested layperson. Only a small minority of families had been able to obtain any written information about their child's condition. Where this had been achieved the information was generally produced by a self-help group, the focus often being on stoma care for babies and young children. In addition, a couple of families referred to the useful-ness of information being disseminated by manufacturers of equipment. One or two families had discovered information in academic textbooks, but even this source was relatively scanty:

'It's sort of a couple of lines in a book.' (*Mother of Neville, 12 years*)

A couple of parents compared this situation unfavourably with the amount of written information which is available when one purchases a piece of household equipment.

'When you have children, you're not given manuals, are you?' (*Mother of Sarah, 11 years*)

'It's like anything else. Instructions for your telly or summat like that ... Sounds stupid! But it's better than finding it out yourself, and blowing it up ... Know what I mean? You don't want to do summat to hurt your kid!' (*Father of Phillip, 9 years*)

While written information about their child's condition was not a high priority for all families, there was evidence that it would have provided a useful supplementary source of infor-mation for some parents, especially in the early stages of their child's life. For example, Stephen's mother reported how much she would have liked someone to say early in her son's life:

'Read this and it will help him a lot.' (*Mother of Stephen, 13 years*)

Language as a factor in communication
'I didn't know that "renal" was kidneys' (mother of Karen, 12 years)

Information needs not only to be timely and accurate, but also intelligible. Sometimes families had been exposed to extensive verbal communication which had conveyed very little to them.

'He was rattling away for half an hour and afterwards, I'm trying to go through it. What did he say about so and so?' (*Mother of Joshua, 11 years*)

'He spoke in riddles anyway. He spoke, he spoke to us medically; and we couldn't understand what he was talking about!' (*Parents of Alex, 11 years, with reference to the doctor at the maternity hospital*)

The non-accessibility of the language used by doctors was a major factor in these mis-communications. The use of medical terms and jargon without explanation was commented upon frequently by families who then felt they had been offered little information, despite having met with doctors who had spent time with them. Technical terms were used inappropriately in the sense that their meaning was unclear to families, parents, as well as children.

'They don't explain the words. They take it for granted you know what they're talking about.' (*Father of Lucy, 8 years*)

'Assuming you're a biologist fanatic, and you know every function of your body, and [they] reel off all this information.' (*Mother of Karen, 12 years*)

A plea for the use of plain English was made by some parents and children.

'Someone who can speak English! Not like hospital crap!' (*Thomas, 11 years*)

'I used to say to them, speak in English to me, don't say it in your language, 'cos your words are far too long.' (*Susan's father, 18 years*)

The importance of communicating in a language which is fully understandable by all those taking part was highlighted by Jane's father. However, his positive experience was atypical as compared to the numbers of families who commented adversely on the type of language used:

'He's a local man, he's a valleys' boy, born in the valleys, and you can sit down to him, you can talk to him. I mean in a common language. And he did give me great, great strength.' (*Father of Jane, now 14 years, of daughter's consultant*)

This emphasis on the central importance of a common language highlights the particular barriers which may face people for whom English is not a first language. These can compound the already isolating impact of this disability. In the previous chapter, a family noted the negative results as regards information about welfare benefits. These effects had a similar impact on information of a medical nature:

> 'Well, going back years . . . my English is getting better every day . . . When I first had him I wasn't aware of any medical terms and the words and things. Over the years I have got used to it and I feel as though I'm very fortunate to have coped with this barrier. I feel as though I'm coming over it. But it must be very difficult for parents who can't understand. You really need to understand. I do sympathise 100 per cent with people with a language barrier. I think there should be some sort of support group for parents like them to understand.' (*Mother of Farooq, 10 years*)

> 'An interpreter would be a start, with information about the condition in Bengali.' (*Parents of Ahmed, 14 years*)

Conclusion
'There's still loads of questions I want to ask' (*mother of Tracey, 16 years*)

The irony that children with a little known and severely disabling condition should be discharged to the care of a parent who has only a very rudimentary grasp of their impairment was brought home to one mother at an outpatient's appointment when her daughter's condition was described in technical terms to a group of medical students.

> 'Here I am, sitting there, thinking "What? Did she have that?" . . . I felt like I was stupid. This was my child he was talking about, and I'd got to take her home with me. And I didn't even know what was wrong with her. He did!' (*Mother of Karen, 12 years*)

The adequacy of information available about this physical impairment and its implications was very variable. Some families' needs were well met, orally at least, and they were very satisfied with their access to the information they needed. Others had experienced major shortfalls, and there was evidence of continuing deficits for some children.

All those working to contribute to the care of children and young people in the study, both professionals and parents, had to cope with an incomplete knowledge base. However, avoidable deficiencies in the information on which families can draw are likely to heighten tension and uncertainty, as well as resulting in errors of approach, both in terms of physical care and in more general management. Ensuring that families have appropriate information available to them is expensive in terms of staff time, and perhaps is not always recognised as a significant but necessary part of treatment. The present emphasis on evaluation of surgeons' performance by quantification of operations performed seems unlikely to encourage the expending of more resources on information giving, although this might well reduce costs in other ways. However, information produced in a variety of media, plus input from specialist nurses, could reduce the amount of time which needs to be spent. Accessible language and the avoidance of negative imagery are important, as is the need for a positive approach which recognises that a good quality of life is possible, even if continence is not achieved.

9. Health and social services: 'We did it on our own basically' (mother of Neville, 12 years)

Neville's mother's view, repeated above, was very commonly expressed by parents when they were asked about service provision. There was a strong feeling of having had to get on with the business of caring for their child. It was very much a parental task, carried out with the minimum of assistance.

'We just got on with it.' (*Parents of Susan, 18 years*)

'I just had to get on with it.' (*Mother of David, 16 years*)

'Just left on your own: get on with it.' (*Mother of Ian, 8 years*)

For some parents there was a feeling of having being left to cope alone with a challenging task and little readily available advice, assistance or support.

'It's all left up to me.' (*Mother of Martin, 10 years, with reference to coping with aftermath of several operations*)

Apart from school, the only major service provider for families was their regional hospital where initial and subsequent surgery was carried out, and reviews of treatment took place.

The key role of Regional Centres
'I just see my consultant. The Health down here don't know much about it' (Stephen, 13 years)

Stephen's comment epitomises the experience of almost all of the families interviewed. It was in the regional and national centres that they learnt to cope with their child's condition and its implications. However, stays in hospital of minimum length and rapid discharge after surgery were the preferred options for children and parents, as well as policy makers and administrators. Thus, families soon found themselves coping at home, very much left to call on their own resources.

'Once they knew I was competent in dilating, that was it. They sent her home.' (*Mother of Sarah, 11 years*)

'"There's the basics of it, get on with it." There was no one. You couldn't fall back on anyone for advice or help, apart from the hospital.' (*Father of Jane, 14 years*)

Parents were aware that they could contact their child's hospital in an emergency. However, about one third of the families did not live within the urban area in which their regional hospital was located, and many of these lived at considerable distances from their hospital. This could add to their sense of isolation.

'If I've any problems I can give her a bell. But Leeds is a long way, isn't it?' (*Mother of Martin, 10 years, of special interest nurse*)

Thus discontent focused on the lack of support and advice available after discharge from hospital.

'I feel the aftercare is lacking.' (*Mother of Josephine, 12 years*)

Learning by trial and error was anxiety-provoking for parents and potentially detrimental to their child. Parents felt they needed more feedback about their performance. Ideally they would have liked someone visiting their homes to offer advice.

'You were shown once and that was it. You got on with it. They need, they should have someone coming.' (*Father of Phillip, 9 years, with reference to colostomy in infancy*)

'If it prolapses or any problems, just got to get there . . . It's the only thing . . . 'Cos no one like, no one comes out to see yer.' (*Mother of Laura, 13 years, regarding ACE procedure*)

The lack of support for these two parents meant they felt very isolated, especially since both were coping without a partner to offer help.

'You feel like no one cares like . . . Just left there, to do it like, sort it all out yourself.' (*Mother of Laura, 13 years*)

'I was beside meself! I mean I was on me own. Running from one end of the cot to the other, seeing to 'em.' (*Father of Phillip, 9 years, describing caring for Phillip and his twin brother when they were toddlers*)

Local Health Services
'Their expertise is limited. Their sort of access to, to any information, that's limited too' (*mother of Karen, 12 years*)

Families soon found they could not expect relevant expertise of this disability in their local primary health care team. General practitioners' experience was such that they could offer little beyond prescriptions for appliances and help with secondary problems.

'Dorothy, you know more about this than I do.' (*Mother of Colin, 8 years, reporting GP's comment*)

'I can't really help you. You are teaching me.' (*Mother of Stephen, 13 years, as above*)

'For all he's brilliant, he sorta said he's like in the Stone Age for Martin's complaint.' (*Mother of Martin, 10 years*)

Health visitors also had little to offer, beyond the support available to families of young, non-disabled children. Parents sometimes found this disappointing since health visitors' nursing training and routine links with families meant they were in a potentially strong position to fulfil the role of listener and advisor with relevant knowledge.

'She was a nice woman, but she didn't know anything, or how to help.' (*Father of Phillip, 9 years*)

'I'd got a fantastic health visitor. She were lovely, but she didn't know what to do.' (*Mother of Joshua, 11 years*)

'She was a waste of space.' (*Mother of George, 14 years*)

Community-based expertise concerning the management of stomas in infants and children seemed to be lacking. In the infrequent event of local stoma nurses being referred to families, they were generally lacking in paediatric experience. The newer and less common ACE procedure was, not surprisingly, even less familiar. Local hospitals too were sometimes not familiar with such developments, so that families were called upon for explanation from their own scanty knowledge base. District nurses were allocated to a few families to carry out specific tasks, usually related to bowel washouts or catheterisation*, and could prove a useful form of support while contact lasted. Contact with continence advisors was reported only rarely, although examples of good practice did exist and one continence advisor had written a booklet explaining the ACE procedure to eight year old Colin.

Children and young people who had no specific management procedure were perhaps the group attracting the least attention and support. With no visible bodily sign of an impairment, they were 'in limbo, sort of thing' (mother of George, 14 years, describing her son's state, prior to a colostomy).

There was much more evidence of goodwill among staff in community services than there was of negative attitudes. Deficits were much more allied to lack of relevant experience, non-availability of accessible reference information and a service delivery system that is not designed to meet the needs of increasing numbers of disabled children with specialised health needs who are living in the community.

Families did cope, but some experienced more problems than others. The rather shady and questionable nature of some of this 'coping' was highlighted by the letter one mother reported that she had written to her daughter's consultant:

'Please, Mr W, we're not coping at the moment, you know, well we are, but we're not.' (*Mother of Susan, 18 years*)

Continence aids
'Sometimes they're good, sometimes they're rubbish' (*mother of George, 14 years, with reference to pads*)

Equipment needed for stomas, ACE and bowel washouts was obtained on prescription, in most cases from general practitioners. Families generally had few problems with this system, although there were some indications of attempts at cost cutting. For example, one family with a fundholding GP were under pressure to reduce the usage and therefore cost of colostomy bags. Where difficulties regarding this type of equipment existed they most commonly related to getting advice about the most suitable type of equipment available, and how best to use it.

Continence pads were needed to some extent by most children in the study, including those utilising the ACE procedure. Their supply to families was rarely totally satisfactory. Firstly nappies were only supplied to babies after the 'pull-through' operation in a few areas, probably because it was assumed that these babies were now functioning like any other. However, in practice families' experience is that 'It's constant diarrhoea' (father of Phillip, 9 years). Hence, the enormous costs and drain on savings indicated in the previous chapter. Moreover, once children were old enough to qualify, families were sometimes not aware of the service and continued to buy their own supplies. Other families bought supplies to supplement their allowance as it was insufficient. Supply was sometimes erratic, as services were reorganised and previously available types of pad withdrawn. 'It used to be murder trying to get them' (mother of Laura, 13 years).

Storage could be a problem, and disposal another. Families did not indicate that any individual assessment of need had been carried out or that their child's preference was a factor taken into account when allocations were made. No family reported that they had been offered pads or pants which were particularly suitable for faecal incontinence. They seemed to be under the impression that there was little choice but to accept the type of pants or pads generally available. Incontinence pads were often of the wrong size.

'They can only do a very small size or a very big size.' (*Mother of Nasreen, 10 years*)

'She was very tiny, and er the pads were humungous. They were so big.' (*Mother of Karen, 12 years*)

Several mothers cut up incontinence pads so as to produce something that fitted their child better, although this could mean they began to disintegrate. The pads' general image also gave problems to school age children, as they had associations with infancy or were intended for elderly adults.

'They had things for elderly people, but not for Susan.' (*Mother of Susan, 18 years*)

'What they give to geriatric patients, you know.' (*Mother of Stephen, 13 years*)

'When we went to collect them they were really like adult nappies! I shouldn't call them that, but incontinence pads. And you couldn't do anything with them. They were horrific.' (*Mother of Josephine, 12 years*)

'He'd like to wear an underpants type of thing. These are just nappies.' (*Mother of Ian, 8 years*)

The visual image that is associated with incontinence pads is particularly important to children and young people. Their privacy is frequently restricted at school. Girls sometimes preferred to use sanitary towels, both because their shape was more discreet and because their discovery in their bags was likely to provoke less comment. However, the slight increase in cost which might arise from supplying more suitable pads or pants would appear to be a worthwhile way of reducing distress to both genders.

Psychological and Psychiatric Services
'To talk about something is better than just to keep it to yourself' (*Simeon, 20 years*)

Some parents and a few young people noted that they had found talking a helpful tool for promoting well-being.

'Talking helps.' (*Mother of Stephen, 13 years*)

'I didn't have anyone to turn to. I couldn't talk to anyone about it. But had someone been available, you know, a shoulder to cry on! A great help!' (*Father of Jane, 14 years*)

Most listeners, insofar as these existed, were close relatives. A very few families had access to a local professional whose listening skills had helped them through a difficult phase. Simeon (20 years) had utilised his GP's counselling skills when depressed, and Colin's mother found her district nurse a sympathetic listener:

'She's always been on the end of the phone when we've had really bad times . . . I've sat and cried for hours on end. And not know where to turn, and she'll come up and have a coffee and make me feel better.' (*Mother of Colin, 8 years, of district nurse*)

Six families had been offered specialist service provision and referred to a psychologist or psychiatrist (see Table 9.1). Families were sometimes rather unclear about the professional status of the personnel involved and about the aim of their input, so that this data should be treated with caution. However, overall the indications are that interventions targeted at helping with secondary problems were valued, but interventions aimed at improving continence failed. Indicative examples are given below.

Table 9.1:   Specialist psychological and psychiatric input

Psychological help from Education Service	Psychiatric ward offered	Psychologist from hospital
2	2 accepted 1 rejected	1

An instance of effective psychological input to overcome secondary problems was reported by Thomas who had received two episodes of counselling. During the first episode, he and his counsellor discussed ways of managing relationships with children at school, including intrusive questioning since he had many anxieties about the potential discovery of his disability. During the second phase of counselling he worked to overcome the distress caused by a traumatic period in hospital. 'She was like, helping a lot' (Thomas, 11 years). There was some evidence of unmet demand for counselling for a few children whose parents felt they needed someone to talk to about their condition and its implications.

By contrast, interventions directed at the incontinence itself did not result in any gains which could be maintained beyond the very short term. Examples of intervention being directed at the incontinence itself were the admissions of Sarah and Faith to what was described as 'a very strict ward' where nurses aimed at changing children's behaviour. Faith hated her three month stay, missing her mother and grandmother and neither she nor her mother understood the reason for her admission. By contrast Sarah enjoyed her six month stay and valued her relationship with the nurses. However, there was no enduring improvement in the continence of either girl. Julie, too, had had a brief hospital admission for toilet training, with the same negative results. None of these three girls had individualised support at school, a service which would probably have proved more useful to them. The offer of admission to a children's psychiatric ward was also proposed for Samuel as a response to his repeated bouts of severe pain. His mother refused this offer, and later the pain was diagnosed as physical in origin.

There was little demand by parents for counselling for themselves, although it was mentioned once or twice with regard to anal and vaginal dilatation. Guidance about management techniques, clear and accurate information and the opportunity to learn from the experience of others were more commonly indicated as being needed. Sarah's mother was unusual in wanting counselling for herself, but her comments are worth recording as they illuminate how family relationships can become distorted. Asked what help she felt she needed, she said:

> 'I think having somebody to talk to, somebody to, to help guide myself. Because obviously I went down a wrong track. In all the blaming myself, blaming Sarah.' (*Mother of Sarah, 11 years*)

Adolescents, teenagers and young adults
'It seems at their age, nobody's bothered, are they?' (*mother of Tracey, 16 years*)

Tracey's mother's view by no means reflected the experience of all of the young people in the study. Robert, for example, who was so enthusiastic about the ACE procedure (see Chapter 3) was 19 years old, and had ongoing contact with his consultant who kept him fully informed of options available. However, several families (largely those with the sons and daughters nearest to adulthood) were either no longer in contact with a hospital about their incontinence or had not been reviewed at their hospital for a long time and were unclear about their next appointment. All of these young people were without a clear management technique which would justify their review by the hospital. However, only one of them had achieved continence and so been clearly discharged.

Sometimes the young people and their parents had given up hope of any improvement, as years of in-patient treatment and out-patient attendance brought no improvement. They had little incentive to push for hospital contact since their contacts resulted in discomfort and disappointment. Several young people reported disappointment as engendered by contact with hospitals which led them to think improvement was possible, only to feel let down later. Thus Simeon (20 years) reported a doctor's anatomical description of him made him feel 'worse in a way', partly because it suggested nothing could be done to help. There are also time costs to be considered in repeated hospital visits and admissions, and the negative effect this can have on school and work.

'It's not very good actually, in school ways. Because you spend so much time in hospital. But most of the time it's just a waste of time being in hospital for it anyway' (*Faith, 17 years*); and subsequently, 'I don't think I'd go to hospital again to have all these things done, because they just don't help at all. I've had so many washouts and enemas, and everything . . . I mean I'm at work now, I don't have time for all these things'.

Young people like this had gradually come to learn that their most satisfactory course was to live with their condition, and while not actually withdrawing from hospital contact, they did not seek it very strenuously. Most of the young people without some clear management technique seemed to have adopted this approach. It was impossible to know whether they had no management procedure because of low amounts of contact with the hospital, or whether their lack of a management procedure which needed review resulted in low hospital contact. However, low amounts of contact meant that these young people lacked access to information about new developments. Very few of these young people knew about the option of the ACE procedure. It was easy to understand why some young people and their families felt disregarded:

'No one's really bothering any more.' (*Karen, 12 years*)

Social services
'There's a stigma attached to social workers' (*mother of Josephine, 12 years*)

Local authority social services departments had a relatively low profile as providers of services to families in the study. The chief reason for contact was advice and support in achieving material improvements in circumstances, usually as the result of claims for disability benefits, as indicated in Chapter 7. Input for this purpose was usually very short-term. A few families had had periods of regular contact for additional reasons, but generally a meeting was specifically focused on financial issues. In some cases families had very positive experiences of social work input. Asked what advice their family would give to other parents in a similar position, Susan's father recommended they get a social worker to help in obtaining entitlements:

''Cos without one of them, you're stumped! . . . You don't know who to write to, or where to write to, or . . . Because it's pointless phoning the benefits' agencies, because, you know . . . they're not very helpful at all.' (*Father of Susan, 18 years*)

Social work assistance was also instrumental in providing help with travel fares to hospital, plus on occasions a telephone or housing adaptations. Social workers also helped with applications to the Family Fund Trust.

'She made an application on our behalf to the Rowntree Fund, and she also got in touch with the people about a downstairs toilet for us.' (*Parents of Alex, 11 years, of their local authority social worker for disabled children*)

Some families did not want contact with social workers, either because they doubted their ability to help or because they were suspicious of them as a result of their high profile role in child protection work. A father who lived in an area where there had been a government inquiry into child protection work in recent years said:

'Ordinary people like me don't trust social workers . . . I've got nowt to hide . . . I've brought these kids up seven and half year, eight year . . . And every ordinary man and woman are suspicious of social workers . . . And they wouldn't tell them owt anyway . . . I've got nowt to hide.' (*Father of Phillip, 9 years*)

As regards child protection work, as already indicated, three families volunteered the information that they had received social work input after incidents where they lost their temper with their child because of the prolonged strain of their incontinence, plus its unmanageable nature. All of the children in question were post 'pull-through', and without any clear management procedure. The two families who received the most contact faced very significant additional problems. They valued the contact they had had, which in each case included a temporary support worker for their affected child.

Despite the recent policy shifts which emphasise the role of the independent sector as a provider of social work services, there was little evidence of voluntary bodies providing supplementary assistance, apart from the highly valued financial support from the Family Fund Trust. As mentioned in the last chapter, self-help groups played a very useful role as regards information, but for a relatively small number of families. Additional contact with a social worker from a voluntary body was reported by one family only. The overall relatively low level of social services' input to these families is probably a reflection of both the generally low priority allocated to social services for physically disabled people, plus the lack of recognition which relates to this particular disability.

Ethnically sensitive services
'It's been a lonely road' (*mother of David, 16 years*)

David's mother's rather poetical reference to 'a lonely road' probably reflects accurately the experience of many families, especially those with older children. It is difficult to say whether it also highlights a sense of isolation compounded by membership of a minority ethnic group.

None of the families from minority ethnic groups felt they had been subject to overt racism by service providers. This view encompassed not only those services alluded to in this chapter, but also those involved in providing education and welfare benefits, as described in Chapters 6 and 7. David's mother considered that she and David had not experienced racism as regards service provision since suitable services had not been available to families of any ethnic group:

'There wasn't much of a service. There was nothing out there.'

In general, this view was consistent with that emerging from the study in that families of all ethnic origins tended to describe the same deficits in service delivery, and describe similar sorts of positive experiences. One hesitates to draw any conclusions from information collected from only five families. However, there is one major area where some minority ethnic families had experienced institutionalised racism and this was in not receiving information in their first language. Access to services was made more difficult and families lacked important knowledge. Ahmed's family's comment on hospital services illustrates this point and how language exacerbates the problems experienced by many families:

'We take him to the hospital but we don't really understand what is going on. I suppose everything is helpful. I am grateful that they try and help him to get better.' (*Father of Ahmed, 14 years*)

Conclusion
'I don't deal with locally. I just deal with Manchester really 'cos Reuben's problems weren't really [understood] round here' (*mother of Reuben, 8 years*)

Parents tended to report a struggle in gaining direct and indirect assistance, feeling they had to fight for what they obtained. This experience of having to battle on behalf of one's disabled son or daughter has been reported before in studies (Baldwin and Carlisle, 1994).

'We had to fight for everything that we wanted, we fought for. Really and truly . . . I mean, I fought to get the pads, I fought to get the incontinence pads, I fought to get the nurse to come into school. I fought for everything.' (*Mother of Joshua, 11 years*)

'I've always felt that I've had to sort of fight, fight for Joel, somehow.' (*Mother of Joel, 14 years*)

There was some evidence within the study of an improvement in services available, in that the least input had been received by the families with the oldest sons and daughters. However, it is difficult to avoid the conclusion that deficits remain. National and regional hospitals play a key and valued role in service provision, but this needs to be provided within the context of other more localised support services.

The experience of these families of feeling left to cope alone is a common one for families of disabled children, including those needing nursing care (Beresford, 1995). Local health service personnel require training about the health needs of disabled children, or at least access to information so that they can offer educated advice. As already indicated, local authorities have a role to play in terms of information about more general support services, including welfare rights, and in helping families to gain access to these services. Improved services in terms of information and support could prevent or limit distress, so that secondary problems would be reduced. Good early support services to parents will produce better parenting of affected children.

Reuben's mother makes clear how services can work together to reduce stress:

'For me, personally, I'm very much somebody who panics and worries, but as soon as somebody says "You have to do this, this, this, this" and it's all laid down without any – Right! I'll get on and do it. But once you're grasping around in the dark, and you don't know what to do – the uncertainty of everything – that's the worrying thing! (Laughs) You could do with somebody saying "Right, there's a leaflet for you to read. And there's this, and I'll come round to your house if you like and have a chat with you. Before you leave hospital, I'll show you how to do a . . .".' (*Mother of Reuben, 8 years*)

10. Conclusion: 'Everybody's got something different about them' (Josephine, 12 years)

This research sought to document the particular experience of children and young people affected by faecal incontinence and that of their families. Its essential message is that this is a distressing disability with wide ranging social implications which are often ignored by service providers. Careful appraisal and effective action is required to minimise the potential danger of further problems developing for the child and their family.

While the information in this report is specific to faecal incontinence, some findings are also strikingly similar to what is known about services to other disabled children and their families. For example, the inadequacy of information available for families of children with a wide range of disabilities is well established (RNIB and Look, 1996; Beresford, 1995; Sloper and Turner, 1992). Moreover, quantitative research has found evidence of high levels of unmet need across the whole population of severely disabled children and young people (Beresford, 1995; Hirst and Baldwin, 1994). A recent report about children with learning disability writes of 'a labyrinth of benefits, therapies and services that must be negotiated' (Mencap, 1997), while a literature review concludes there is a need for 'establishing service priorities and clear criteria for receipt of services' (Baldwin and Carlisle, 1994). Thus the families participating in the study shared with other families of disabled children a common experience of social disadvantage which is not countered effectively by the services which are on offer. Services are insufficiently user-friendly, not distributed in an even-handed fashion and inconsistently available across England and Wales.

The final chapter to this report concludes by exploring two further experiences which children and young people with physically induced faecal incontinence have in common with some other disabled people. These themes are the life-threatening nature of the original impairment, and the physical pain which may be associated with faecal incontinence. Although not specifically asked about these aspects of their son's or daughter's condition, families made frequent reference to them and they are included here as a significant part of their experience. The report ends with the views of the children and young people about what they have learnt from their disability. Their comments reinforce the need for society's acceptance of difference.

A life-threatening impairment
'Our Tom says "I'm glad you didn't die"' (Tracey, 16 years)

During their account of their birth and early years, parents frequently referred to the life-threatening nature of their son's or daughter's original impairment. An oblique message of this fact had often been communicated to them when nurses or medical staff wanted a name for the child very soon after disclosing discovery of the bowel impairment. This was in preparation for an early baptism. The implications of the child's condition were also communicated more directly.

> 'I think they put it in your mind that here's a very poorly child . . . You know: "Don't be disappointed if she dies."' (*Mother of Megan, 12 years*)

> 'I said "She's not going to die, she's not going to die, is she?" And he said "Well, medicine's not a hundred per cent, and I can't give you that guarantee."' (*Mother of Karen, 12 years, describing conversation with hospital doctor*)

The children and young people interviewed mentioned the life-threatening nature of their impairment more rarely, like Tracey quoted above, or Simeon who said of his consultant:

> 'Of course I can't blame him for not teaching me anything about the problem, because he saved my life in the first place. So I owe him the fullest respect really.' (*Simeon, 20 years*)

Pain
'Physical things and mental things. Just pain in every sort of way' (*Thomas, 11 years*)

Children and young people were asked what they never wanted to experience again. Their replies almost always referred to some experience related to their condition rather than any other aspect of their lives. Sometimes the experience had an obviously social aspect, of the type which has been referred to earlier in the report:

> 'Junior school, swimming lessons, being picked on.' (*Robert, 19 years*)

Incidents of soiling were often mentioned, as were physical management techniques:

> 'Colostomy, definitely.' (*Josephine, 12 years*)

> 'Washouts and enemas and things like that.' (*Faith, 17 years*)

> 'Going through what I've gone through with Gilbert.' (*Susan, 18 years, who calls her colostomy 'Gilbert'*)

For a substantial number of the children and young people, hospital admissions along with surgery and anaesthesia were the experiences they least wanted to repeat. Most of the children and young people in the study had been admitted to hospital on several occasions and almost all had undergone surgery more than once, some many times. It would be easy, therefore, to underestimate the trauma of hospital stays, and operations in particular. Children reported worrying acutely about them, and their parents sometimes reported that they were aware this was the case. However familiar the hospital was and however competent the staff, children often found it a very anxiety-provoking environment.

> 'I hate getting tubes up my nose and I had to have one up and I was worried about that.' (*Laura, 13 years, describing concerns prior to operation for ACE*)

While some parents expressed pride in how well their son or daughter had dealt with the hospital admissions and surgery, the children themselves would have preferred to be without them, as they knew their non-disabled peers were. These considerations sometimes led to their expressions of a desire to be non-disabled.

'I wish I'd been born normal. I wish I didn't have all these problems.' (*Reuben, 8 years, as reported by his mother. Reuben is awaiting further major surgery.*)

Learning from disability
'I have learnt to listen more to other people who have problems' (*Nasreen, 10 years*)

The children and young people in the study were asked what they had learnt from coping with their disability. The thoughts of some turned to concrete skills in dealing with procedures and equipment. Some felt they had learnt how much adversity they could cope with and this emphasised their strengths to them.

'I think it's made me stronger . . . Well, if I can cope with this . . . I can cope with anything else.' (*Laura, 13 years*)

'I can cope with anything really . . . Now if I get them (i.e. severe abdominal pains) again, I know how to cope and all that . . . So, if I get the pain again, like you've gotta, you've gotta cope with it, I think. It's learning a lot, isn't it?' (*Samuel, 13 years*)

The children and young people were aware at first hand of how it feels to face pain and prejudice. Through their own experiences at school and elsewhere, the children had learnt that everyone was entitled to respect.

'I've been through it so I should respect others who have experienced the same or different.' (*Megan, 12 years*)

'Not to skit people or make fun of people, who've got such and such a problem.' (*Patrick, 12 years*)

Some of the children and young people interviewed felt they had learnt to understand how other people might feel and to have concern for them. This view expressed by affected children and young people was supported by the fact that several parents also spontaneously mentioned this tendency in their affected son or daughter. This sort of empathic behaviour has been reported before in research about disabled children (see Eiser, 1993).

'I've learnt to understand other people's problems . . . and just because they've got something wrong with them, it doesn't mean they're different.' (*Faith, 17 years*)

'I feel I can relate to people who have problems and that I can really empathise with them.' (*Haroon, 22 years*)

This breadth of experience had encouraged some young people to begin to reflect on the diversity of human experience, and on the nature of 'difference', a word which was used by several children.

'Everybody's got something different about them, and some things are just more different than others. But we're all – I don't know – different in different ways.' (*Josephine, 12 years*)

Appendix

Methods

Data were collected from 35 families with a son or daughter who was born with imperforate anus. Thirty-one of these were contacted via the Family Fund Trust Database; this response was from a total of 48 families approached. A self-help group and special interest nurses assisted with the remaining contacts. Affected children in 11 families were attending primary school; the sons and daughters of the remaining families were at secondary school or of working age.

Potential families were first informed about the study by an information leaflet. Those who indicated active interest in participating were contacted by telephone for further discussion. Parents gave written consent to the interviews, as did the children and young people who took part. Thirty-one children and young people were interviewed as part of the study, the remainder preferring not to do so. Information was collected from parents only, in these four families. Mothers were considered chief carers (sometimes jointly with their partner) by all but two families in which the fathers were lone parents. The usual pattern of interviewing was that the chief carer or carers provided information first, and then young people gave their views independently afterwards.

However, sometimes parents and children chose to participate together, or it was preferred that a parent should be present when their child was interviewed. Semi-structured interview schedules were employed with both children and carers. Interviews which took place in families' own homes were routinely taped and transcribed, except on the few occasions where families wanted notes to be taken.

Special efforts were made to include the views of families from minority ethnic groups. The prevalence of imperforate anus in people from minority ethnic groups in England and Wales is thought to be commonest among people originating from the Indian sub-continent. The experience of the study supports this view, and four of the five minority ethnic families who contributed to the study were Muslim. They were interviewed by Robinah Shah, who also acted as an advisor to the project.

Analysis was carried out by the framework method. This involved a 'systematic process of sifting, charting and sorting material according to key issues and themes' (Ritchie and Spencer, 1994, p 177). General advice, support and feedback about the study was given by two teenagers and two young adults who have personal experience of faecal incontinence. This was additional to that received from an advisory body of professional and parent members.

Glossary

ACE
> This stands for antegrade continence enemas. The enemas are delivered by *catheter* in an antegrade fashion – that is, from the top of the colon to the rectum. The enemas are delivered through the appendix, one end of which is brought onto the skin to the right and below the tummy button. If the appendix has been removed, other methods are available.

Bowel washout
> The process whereby a large *catheter* is inserted into the rectum and the rectum then washed clean through the catheter using large quantities of fluid. Also known as rectal washout and colonic irrigation.

Catheter
> 'A flexible tube for insertion into a narrow opening so that fluids may be introduced or removed'. (*Oxford Concise Medical Dictionary, 1994*)

Catheterisation
> Insertion of *catheter*, in this context usually for *ACE* procedure or *bowel washout*.

Colostomy
> 'Surgical operation in which a part of the colon is brought through the abdominal wall and opened in order to drain or decompress the intestine. The part of the colon chosen depends on the site of obstruction . . . The colostomy may be temporary, eventually being closed after weeks or months to restore continuity; or permanent, usually when the rectum or lower colon has been removed. An appliance is usually worn over the colostomy opening (see *Stoma*) to prevent soiling the clothes'. (*Oxford Concise Medical Dictionary, 1994*)

Dilatation

'The enlargement or expansion of a hollow organ or cavity'. (*Oxford Concise Medical Dictionary, 1994*) In the context of this research, dilators were usually metal or glass rods, sometimes supplied in sets graduated in size. They are inserted into the anus (or occasionally the vagina) to prevent narrowing, most commonly after surgery.

Family Fund Trust

Formerly known as the Family Fund, this is an independent organisation which 'is funded by the Department of Health. The Trust's purpose is to ease the stress on families who care for very severely disabled children under 16, by providing grants and information related to the care of the child'. (Family Fund Trust, 1996) (Address: PO Box 50, York YO1 2ZX)

Family Fund Trust Database

Computer record of all families registered with the Family Fund Trust. The database holds details of families with one or more disabled child who have applied to the Family Fund Trust since 1973.

Hidden disability

See *Invisible disability*.

Hirschsprung's Disease

A congenital condition in which the anal sphincter, the rectum and sometimes a variable length of bowel have failed to develop a normal nerve network. Continence problems may persist after surgery, including constipation and over-flow diarrhoea.

Imperforate anus

'Partial or complete obstruction of the anus; a condition, discovered at birth, due to failure of the anus to develop normally in the embryo. There are several different types . . . If the defect is extensive a temporary opening is made in the colon (see *Colostomy*) with later surgical reconstruction of the rectum and anus'. (*Oxford Concise Medical Dictionary, 1994*)

Invisible disability

An invisible disability is one which is not obvious to an outside observer (autism or epilepsy are well known examples). While people with an invisible (or hidden) disability escape the automatic devaluation which is reported by people with a disability obvious to the casual observer, social expectations of them are inappropriate, being either difficult or impossible for them to fulfil.

Ostomy

'Surgical opening into an organ or part. Example: colostomy (into the colon)'. (*Oxford Concise Medical Dictionary, 1994*)

Pull-through

The generic term applied to a group of operations whereby bowel is brought to the skin to form an anus and rectum not present at birth.

Self-help group

People and families affected by a similar condition or set of circumstances who form a group to promote mutual support and information sharing. For example, NASPCS (tel. 01560 322024) is a registered charity for incontinent and ostomy children, and the GMD Support Network (tel. 01799 520580) focuses on those with gut motility disorders. Contact-a-Family (tel. 0171 383 3555) can provide more details about these and other self-help groups.

Sphincter

A ring of muscle that surrounds an opening on the body, and which can contract.

Spina bifida

A developmental defect in the newborn baby where one or more vertebrae have failed to close over the spinal cord. The lesion may be open or closed. Incontinence may be associated with this condition.

Statement of Special Educational Need

This may be issued by a Local Education Authority after a formal assessment so that individual children with serious difficulties are allocated additional staff time and resources. Rights of parents in this regard were increased by the Education Act, 1993.

Stoma

'The artificial opening of a tube (for example, colon or ileum) that has been brought to the abdominal surface'. (*Oxford Concise Medical Dictionary, 1994*)

Urostomy

Surgical creation of an opening from the ureter, which carries urine from kidney.

References

Baldwin, S and Carlisle, J (1994) *Social Support for Disabled Children and their Families. A Review of the Literature*. HMSO

Beresford, B (1994) *Positively Parents. Caring for a Severely Disabled Child*. HMSO

Beresford, B (1995) *Expert Opinions. A National Survey of Parents Caring for a Severely Disabled Child*. Polity Press

Bibby, P and Lunt, I (1996) *Working for Children. Securing Provision for Children with Special Educational Needs*. David Fulton Publishers

Bone, M and Meltzer, H (1989) *The Prevalence of Disability Among Children: Report 3*. HMSO

Buchanan, A (1992) *Children who Soil. Assessment and Treatment*. John Wiley

Diseth, T and others (1994) 'A psychosocial follow-up of ten adolescents with low anorectal malformation', *Acta Paediatric*, **83**, 216–21

Dittesheim, J and Templeton, J (1987) 'Short term and long term quality of life in children following the repair of high imperforate anus', *Journal of Pediatric Surgery*, **XXII**, 7, 581–7

Eiser, C (1993) *Growing up with a Chronic Disease*. Jessica Kingsley Publishers

Ginn-Pease, M E and others (1991) 'Psychological adjustment and physical growth in children with imperforate anus or abdominal wall defects', *Journal of Pediatric Surgery*, **XXVI**, 9, 1129–35.

Hirst, M and Baldwin, S (1994) *Unequal Opportunities. Growing Up Disabled*. HMSO

Latham, R and Matthews, W (*eds*) (1995) *The Diary of Samuel Pepys*. Harper Collins

Ludman, L and Spitz, L (1996) 'Coping strategies of children with faecal incontinence', *Journal of Pediatric Surgery*, **XXXI**, 4, 563–7

Ludman, L, Spitz, L and Kiely, E M (1994) 'Social and emotional impact of faecal incontinence following surgery for anorectal anomalies', *Arch Dis Child*, **71**, 194–200

MENCAP (1997) *Left in the Dark*. MENCAP

Oliver, M (1990) *The Politics of Disablement*. Macmillan

Ritchie, J and Spencer, L (1994) 'Qualitative data analysis for applied policy research' *in* Bryman, R and Burgess, R G *Analyzing Qualitative Data*. Routledge

RNIB and Look (1996) *What Families Need Now. A Report of the Needs of Families with Visually Impaired Children in Scotland.* RNIB and Look

Sloper, P and Turner, S (1992) 'Service needs of families with children with severe physical disability', *Child Care, Health & Development*, **18**, 250–82

Thomas, A, Bax, M and Smyth, D (1989) *Health and Social Needs of Young Adults with Physical Disabilities.* McKeith Press

Touloukian, R J (1969) 'Management of the newborn with imperforate anus', *Clinical Paediatric (Phila)*, **8**, 38

Index